MW01452734

My Pregnancy JOURNAL

My *Pregnancy* JOURNAL

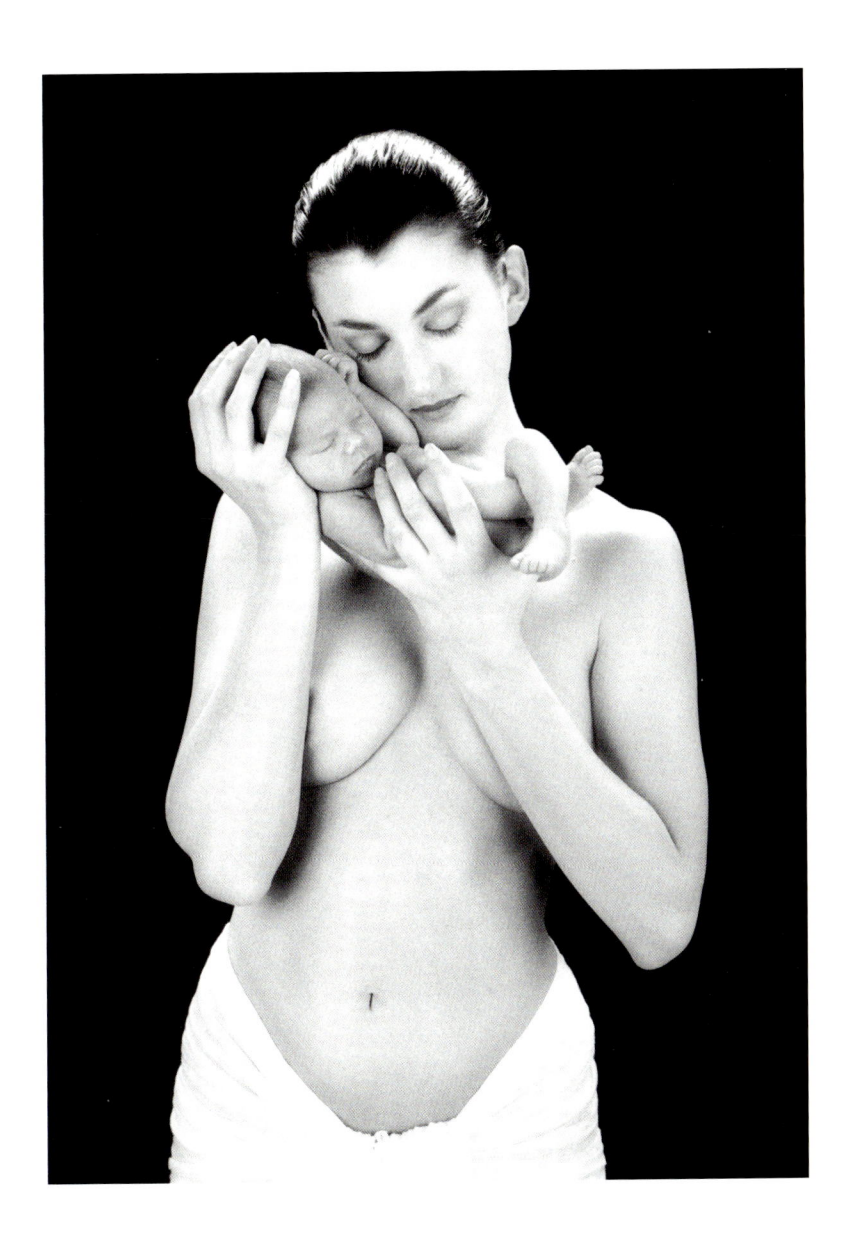

ANNE GEDDES

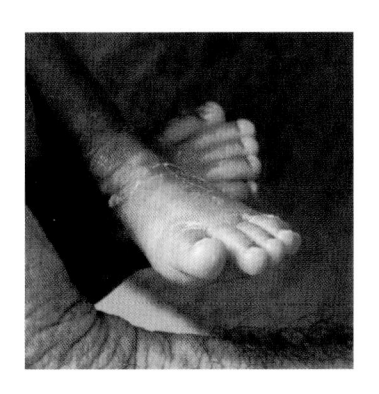

My Pregnancy Journal
by

....

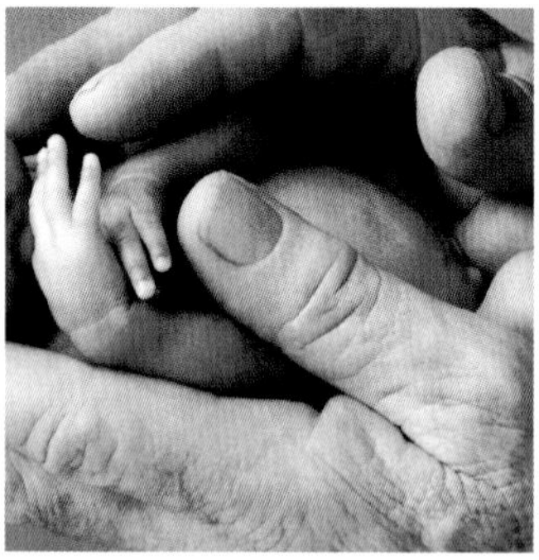

- FINDING OUT -

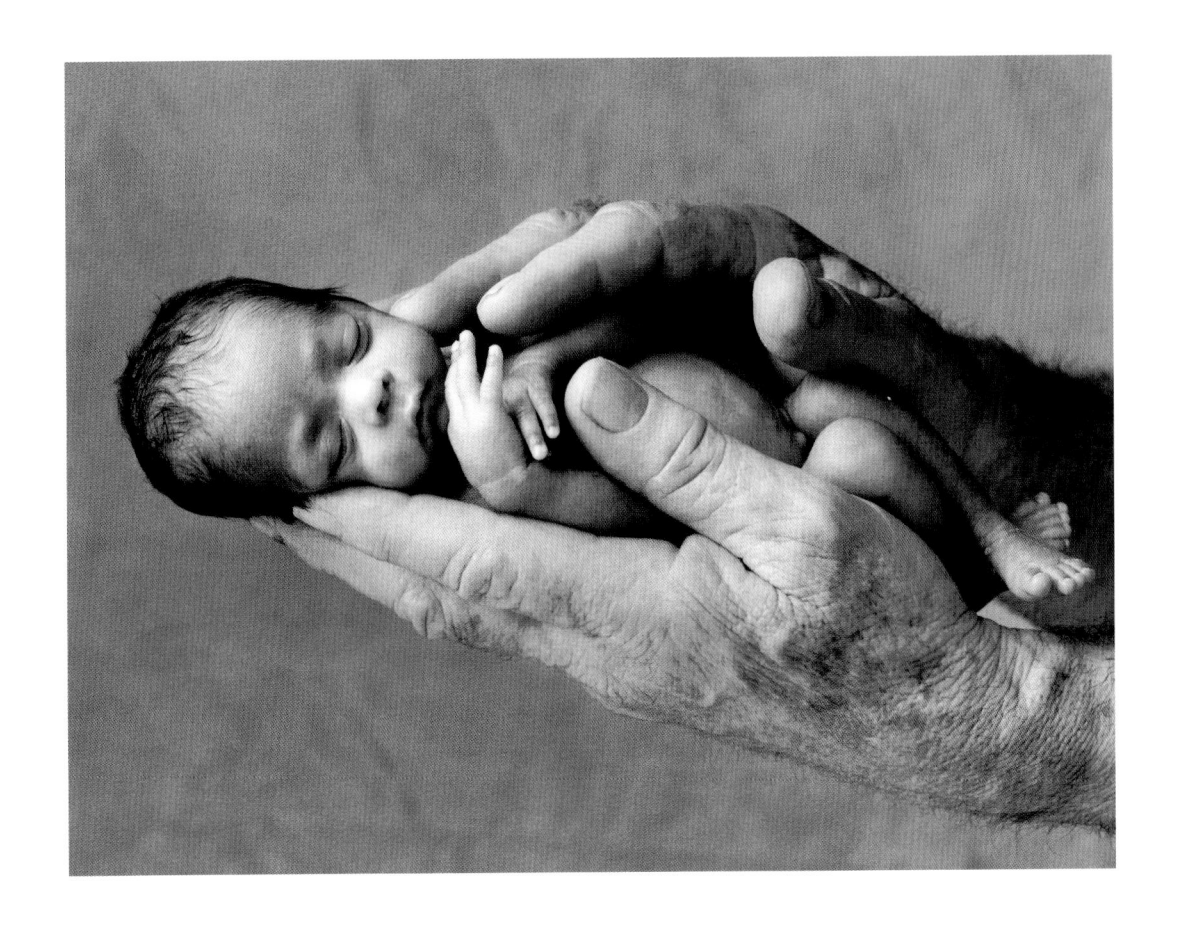

- FINDING OUT -

Baby's due date

I thought I might be pregnant because

- FINDING OUT -

How I felt when the pregnancy was confirmed

Who was with me at the time

- FINDING OUT -

Who I shared the news with first ... Their reaction

- FINDING OUT -

Reaction of family and friends to the news

- FIRST THINGS FIRST -

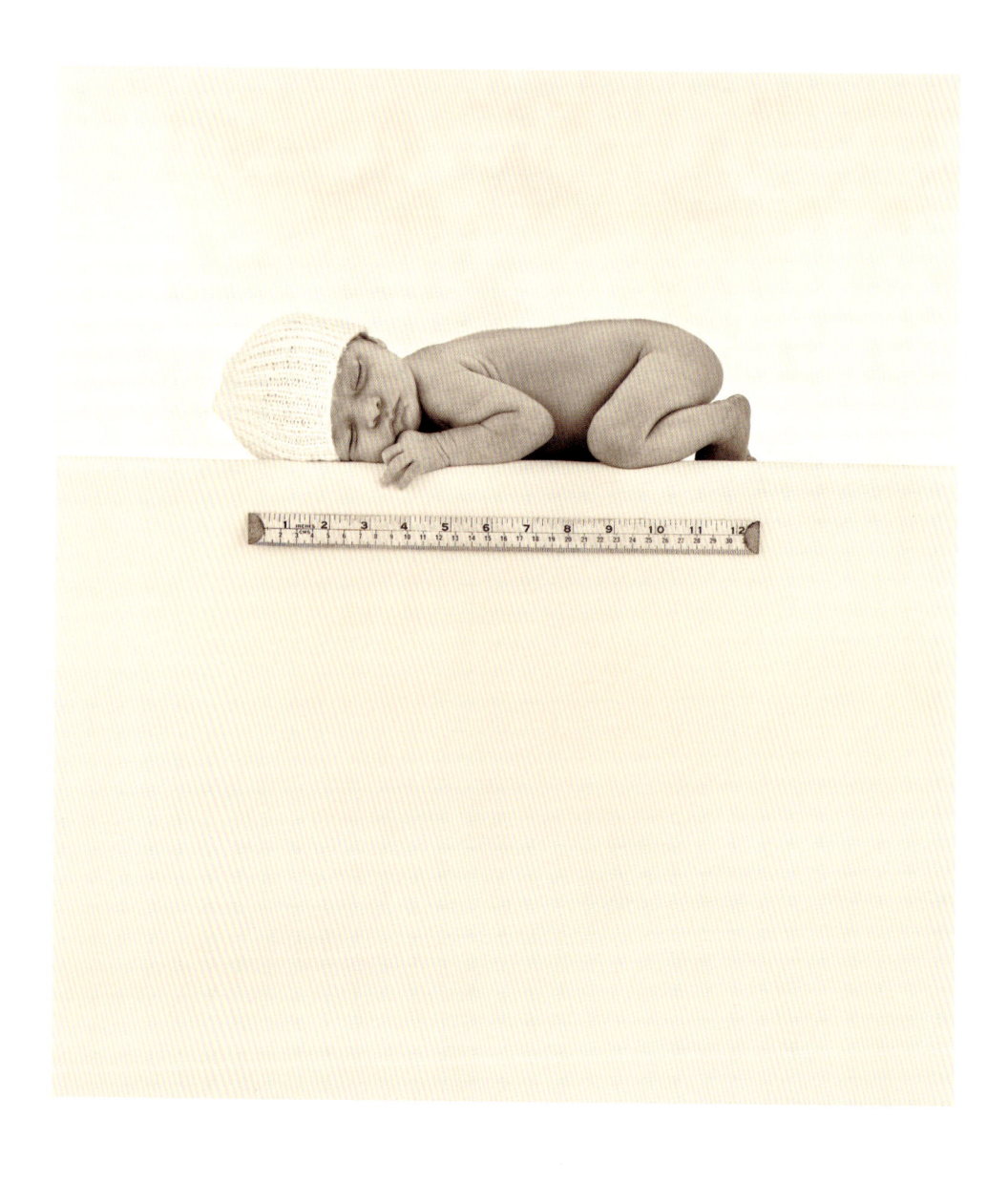

Where I would like to give birth

I chose ... as my caregiver because

- FEELINGS ABOUT BECOMING A MOTHER -

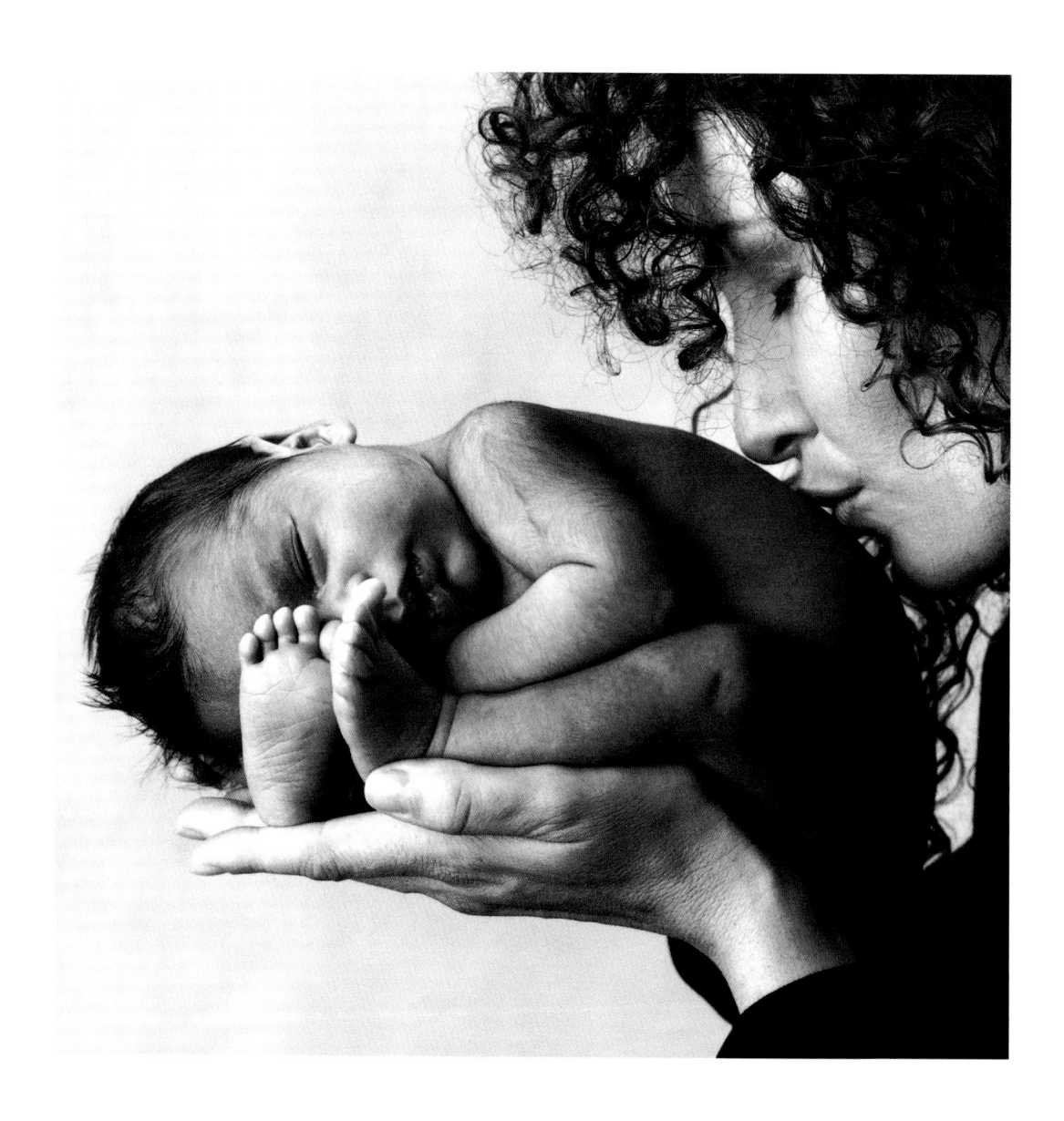

*My thoughts
on motherhood*

*My thoughts
on childhood*

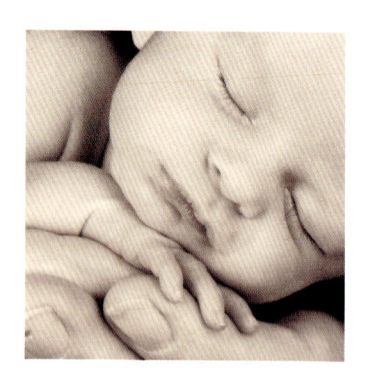

The First
THREE MONTHS

The First
THREE MONTHS

- JOURNEY THROUGH PREGNANCY -

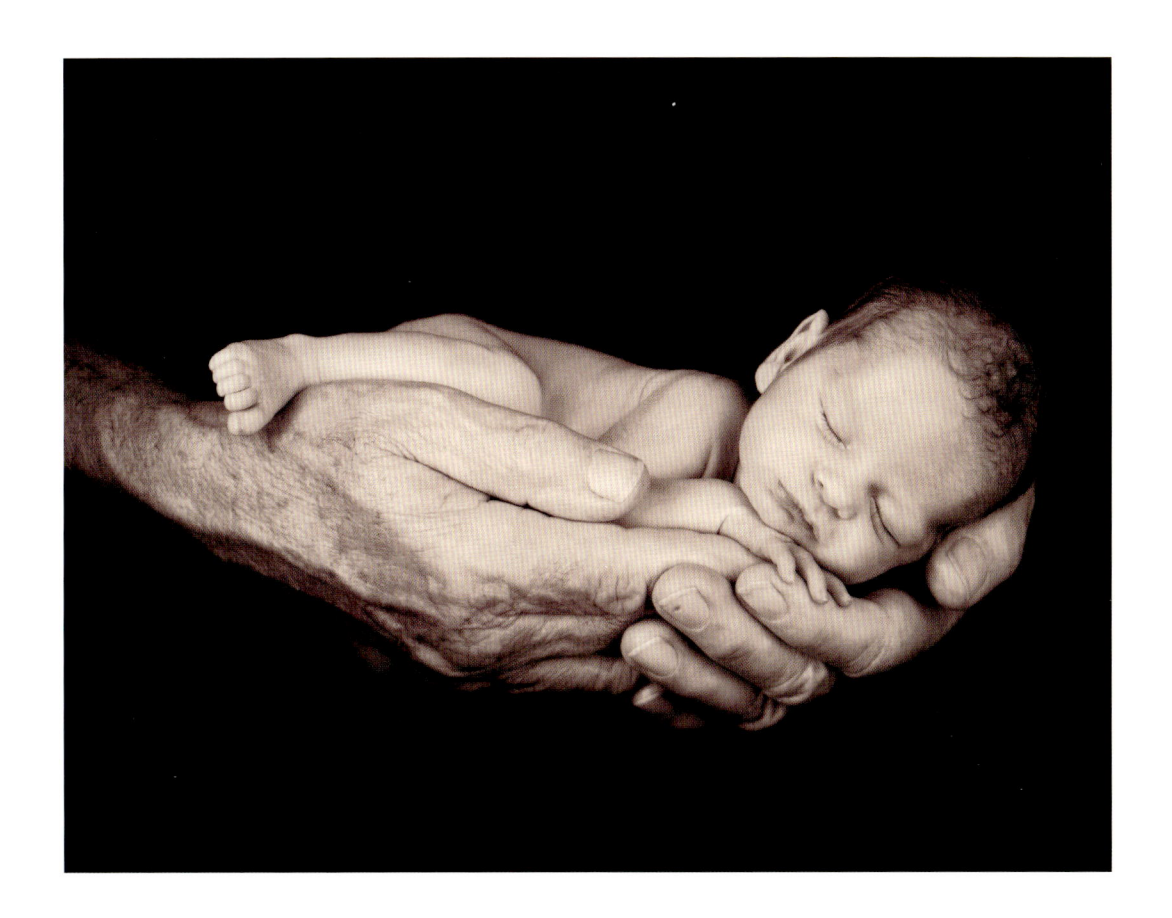

- JOURNEY THROUGH PREGNANCY -

Changes I have noticed about my body

- JOURNEY THROUGH PREGNANCY -

My food preferences

Foods and drinks I cannot tolerate

- JOURNEY THROUGH PREGNANCY -

I am excited about

- JOURNEY THROUGH PREGNANCY -

I am feeling anxious about

- GOOD ADVICE -

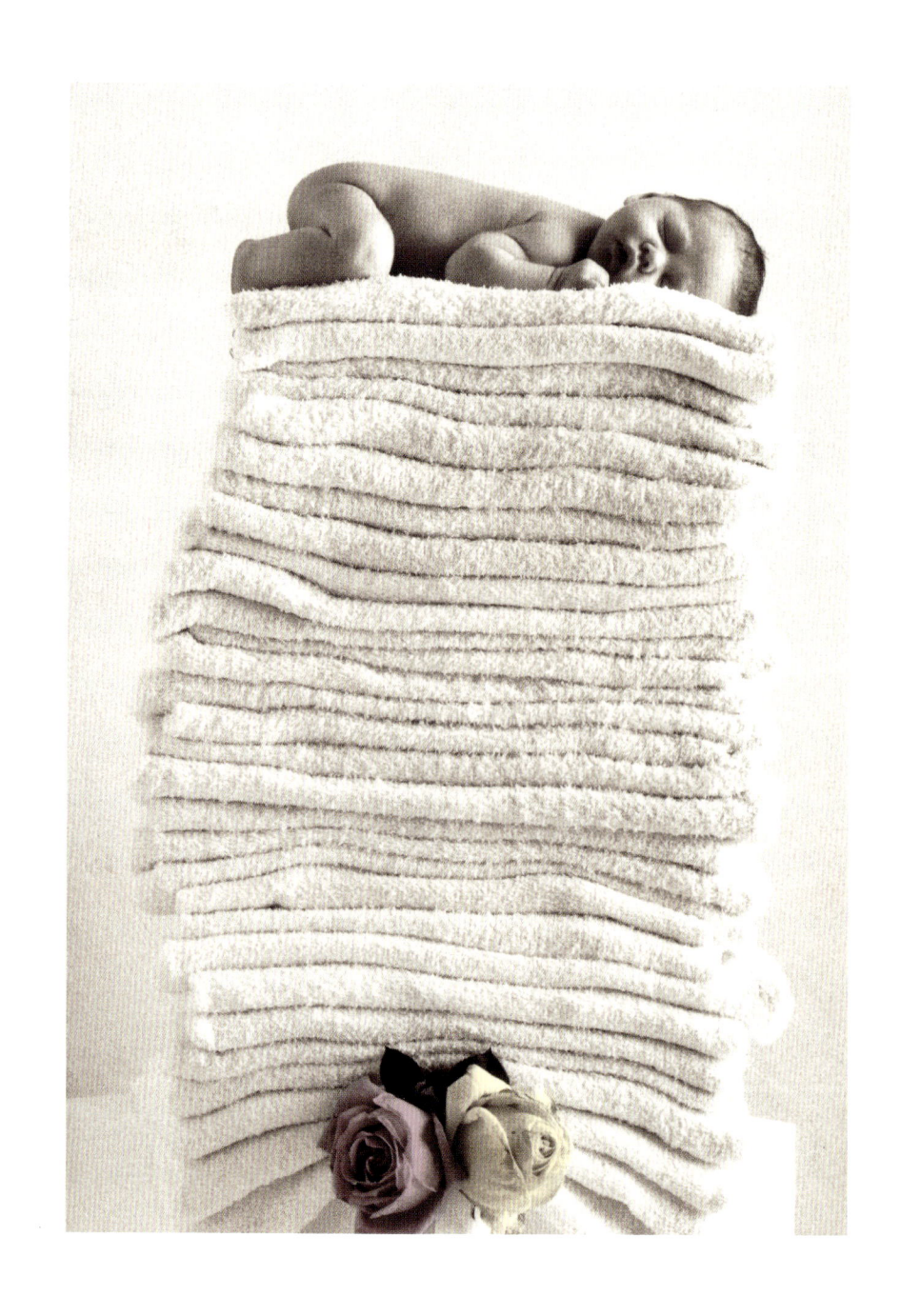

Interesting things I have learned or been told by others

Some good advice I received from ... was

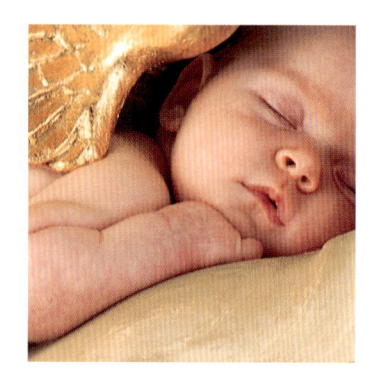

The Second
THREE MONTHS

The Second
THREE MONTHS

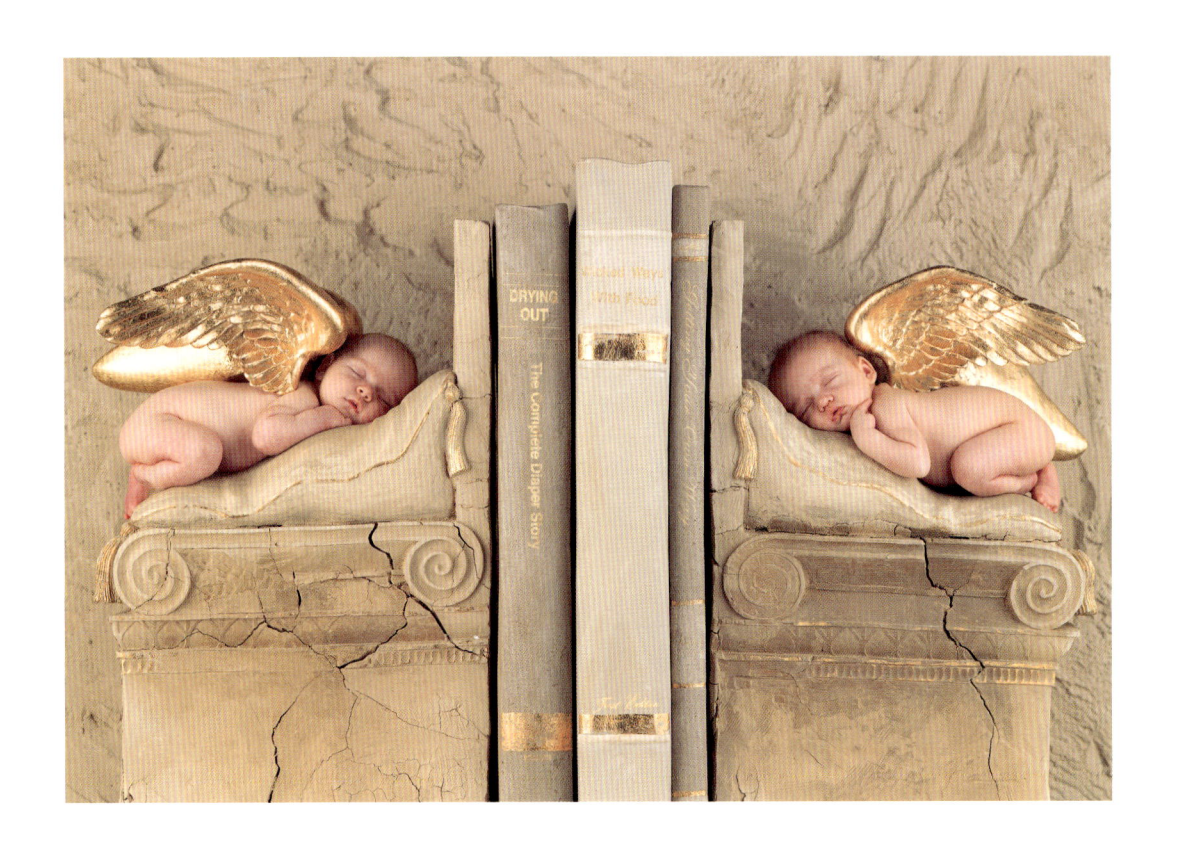

- MY DISAPPEARING WAISTLINE -

- MY DISAPPEARING WAISTLINE -

What I am really enjoying about being pregnant

But this isn't much fun

- MY DISAPPEARING WAISTLINE -

Changes I have noticed about my body

- FIRST LOOK -

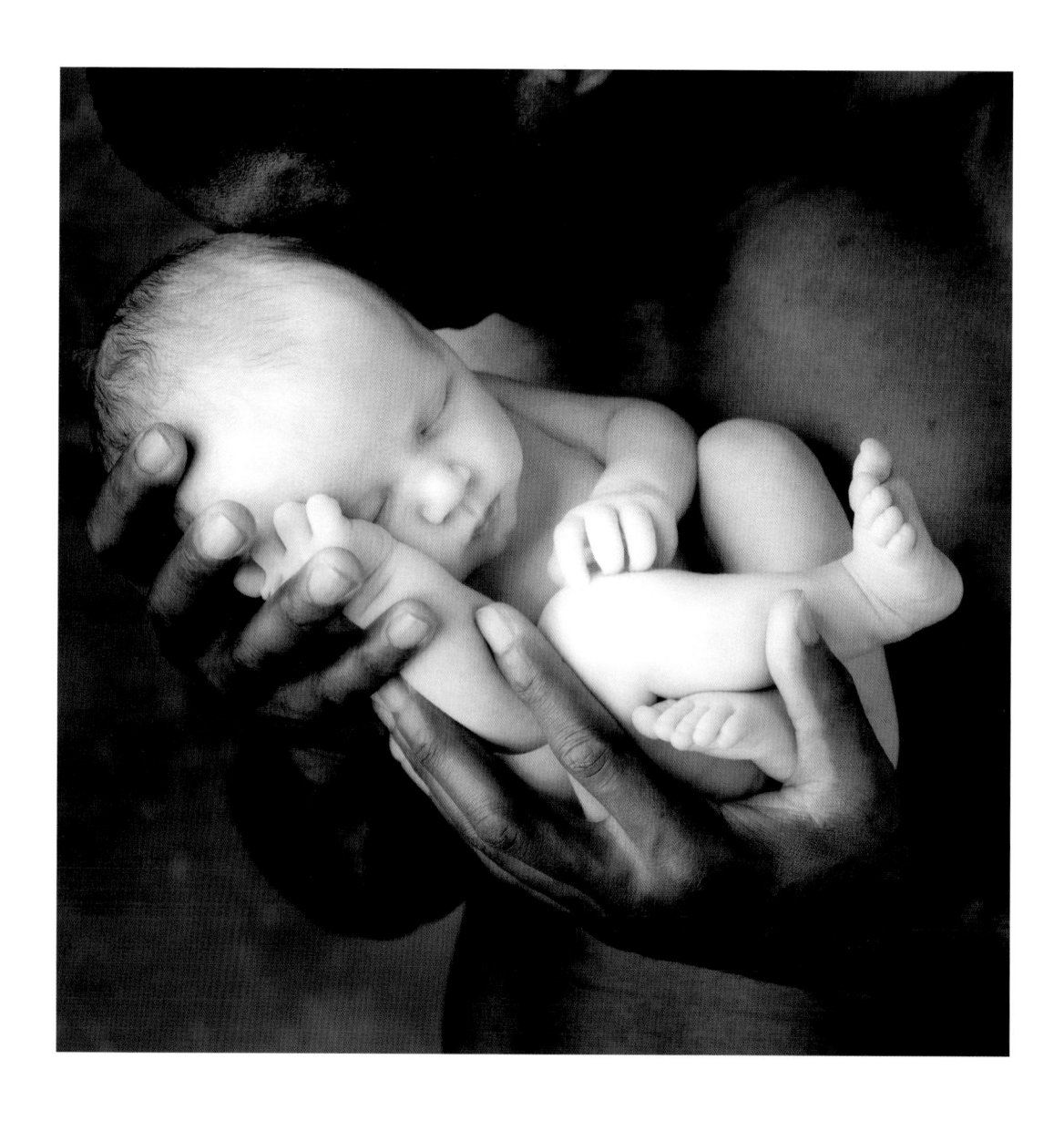

My first ultrasound was ... at

How I felt about the ultrasound

- FIRST LOOK -

I wanted to know the sex of my baby because

- FIRST LOOK -

I did not want to know the sex of my baby because

A SPECIAL NOTE TO MY BABY -

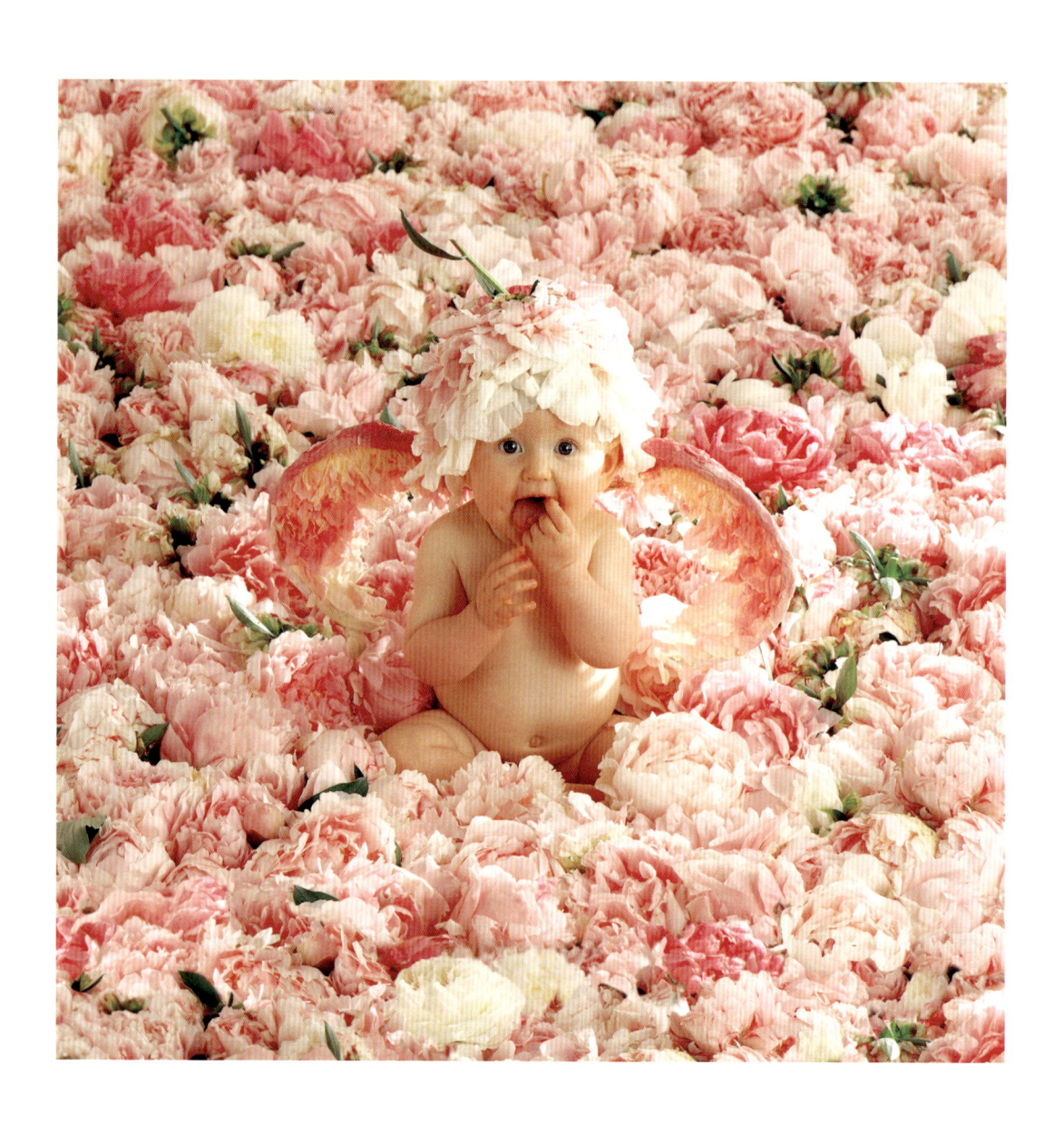

*I have been
thinking about*

*I would like
you to know*

- BABY'S FIRST MOVEMENTS -

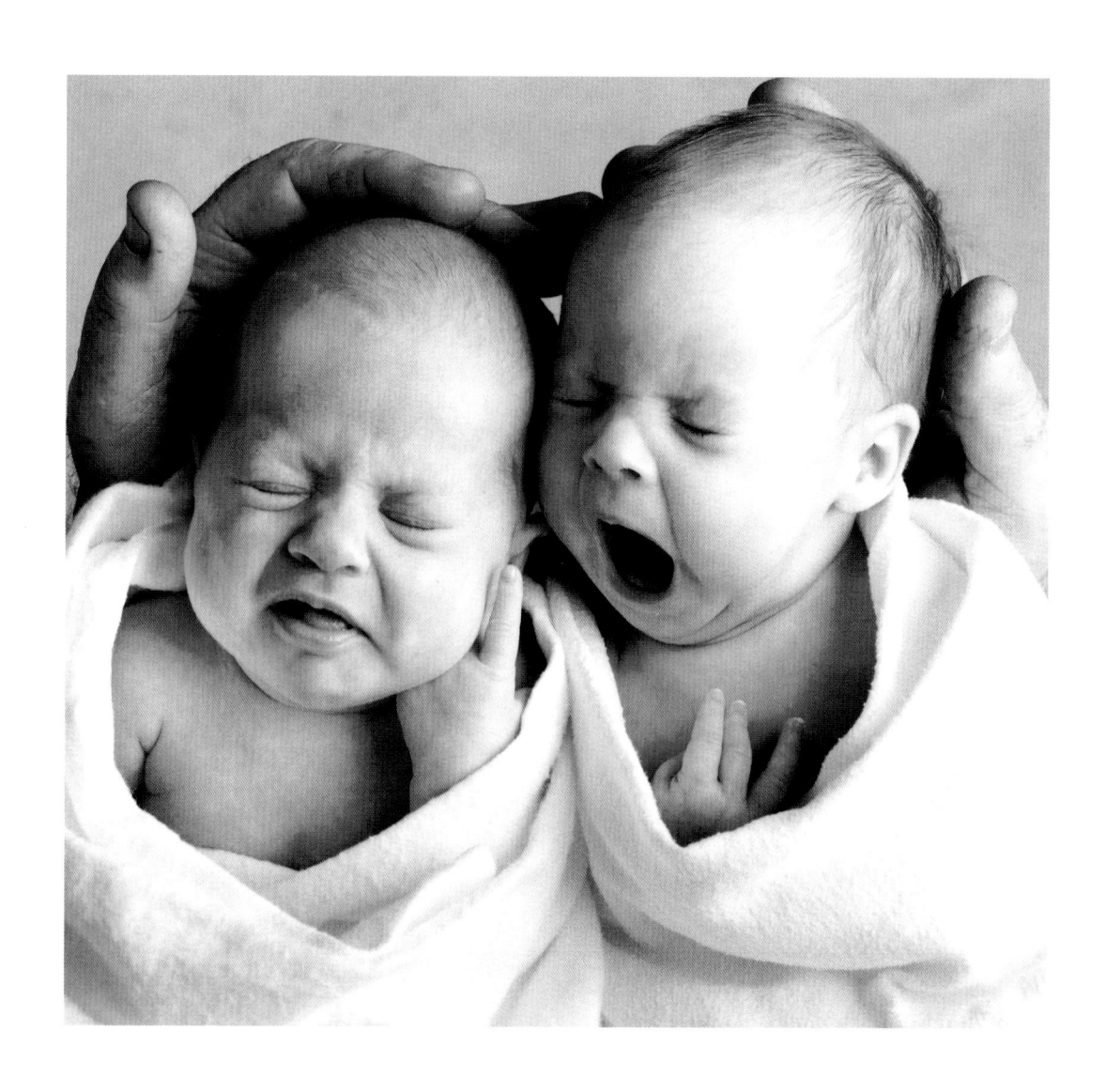

*I first felt my
baby move . . .
It felt like*

*How long it
was before
someone else
could feel my
baby move*

- WHAT'S AHEAD -

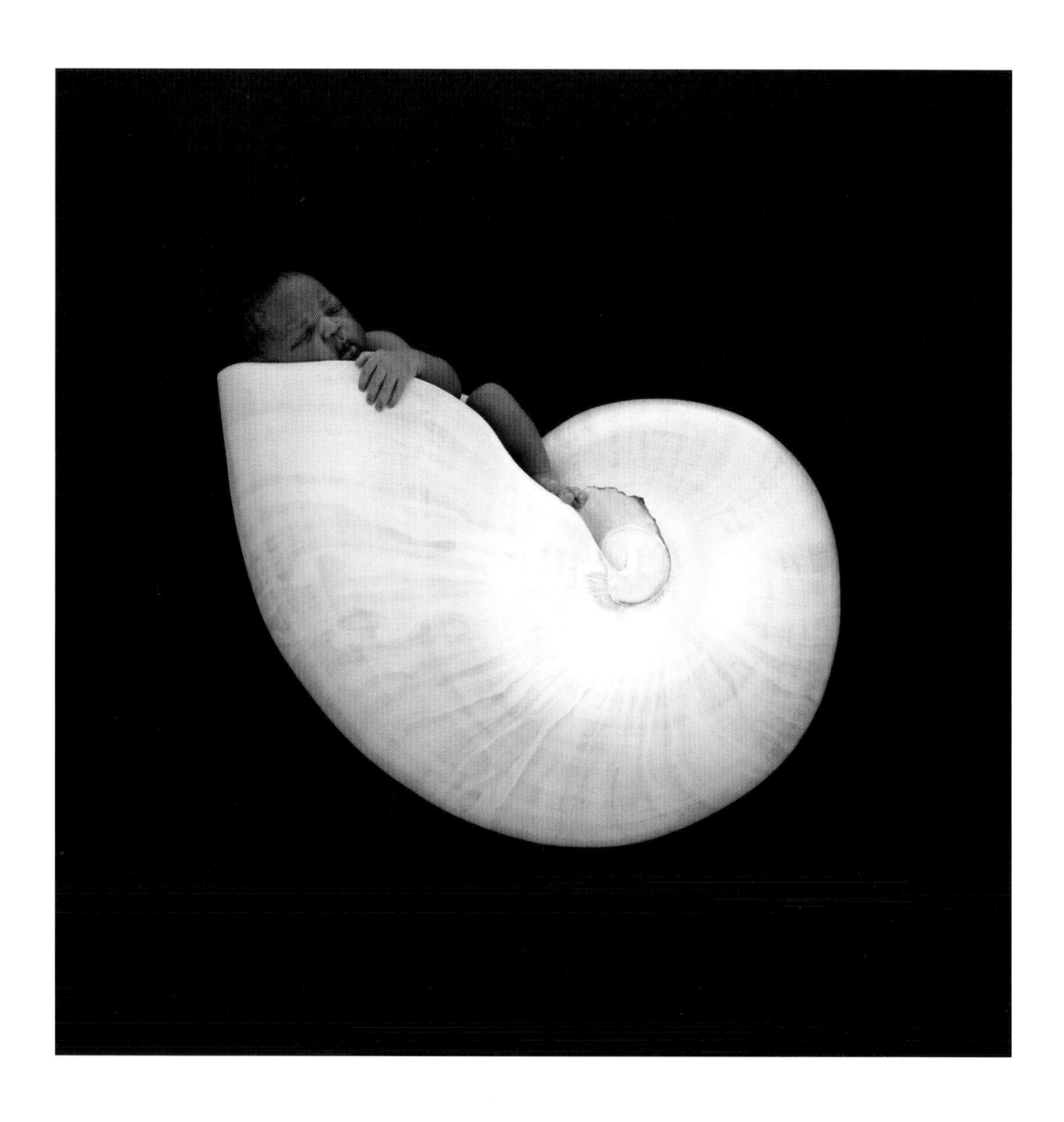

I am attending childbirth classes at

Useful information

- KEEPING UP -

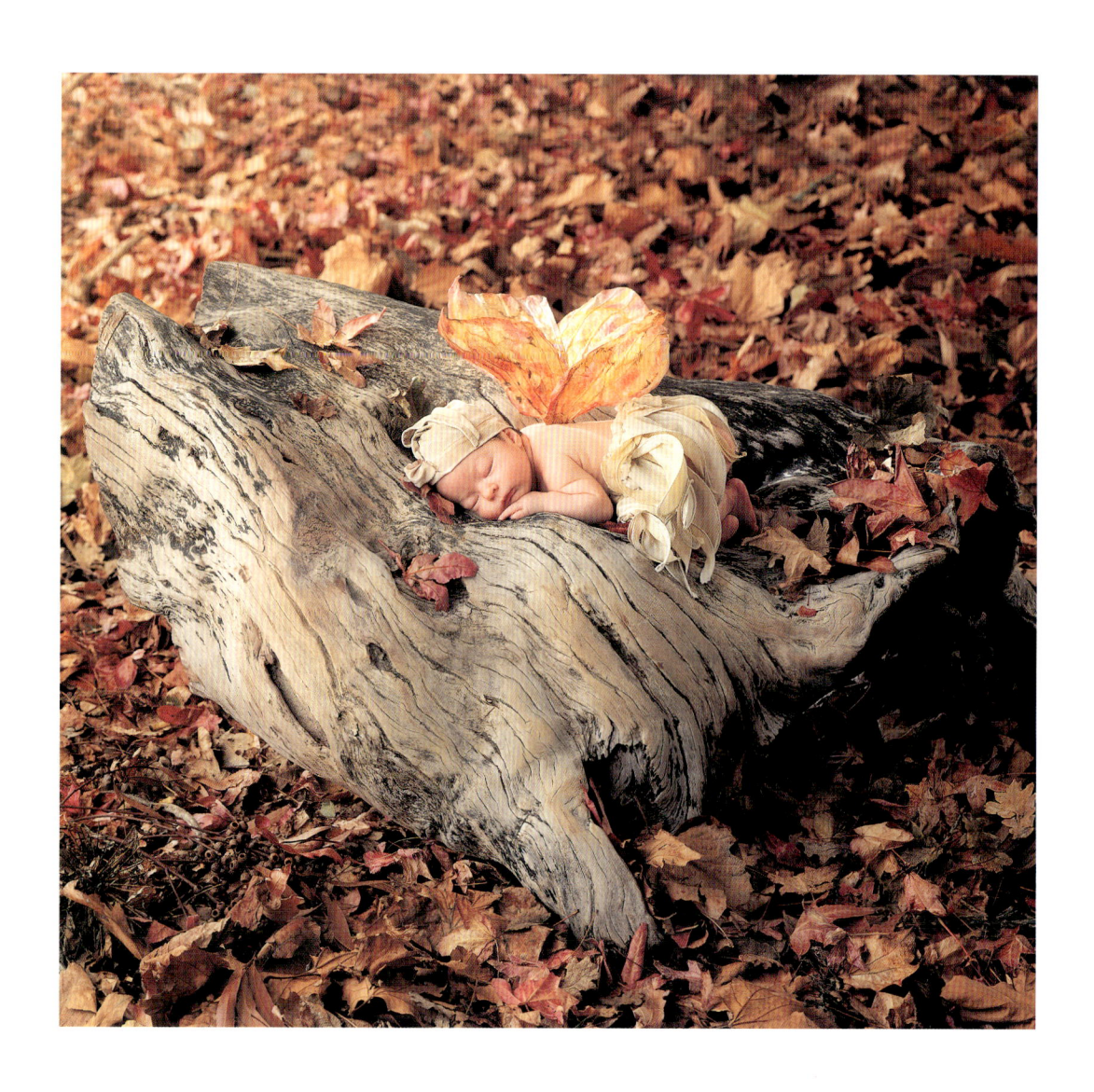

Comments about my visits to my caregiver

- CHANGING RELATIONSHIPS -

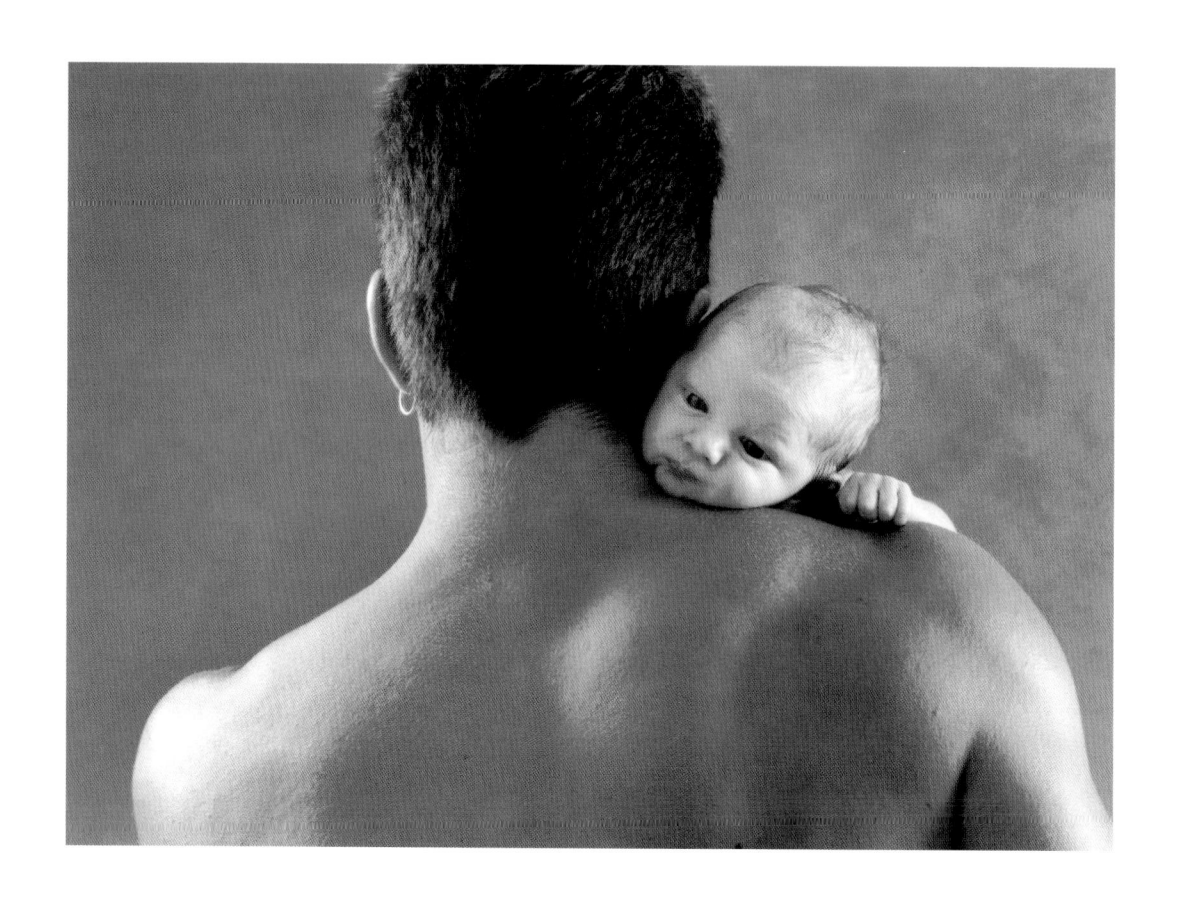

How being pregnant has changed my relationship with those close to me

- CHANGING RELATIONSHIPS -

How being pregnant is different from what I expected

- CHANGING RELATIONSHIPS -

How I am feeling about myself and being pregnant

- SPECIAL MOMENTS -

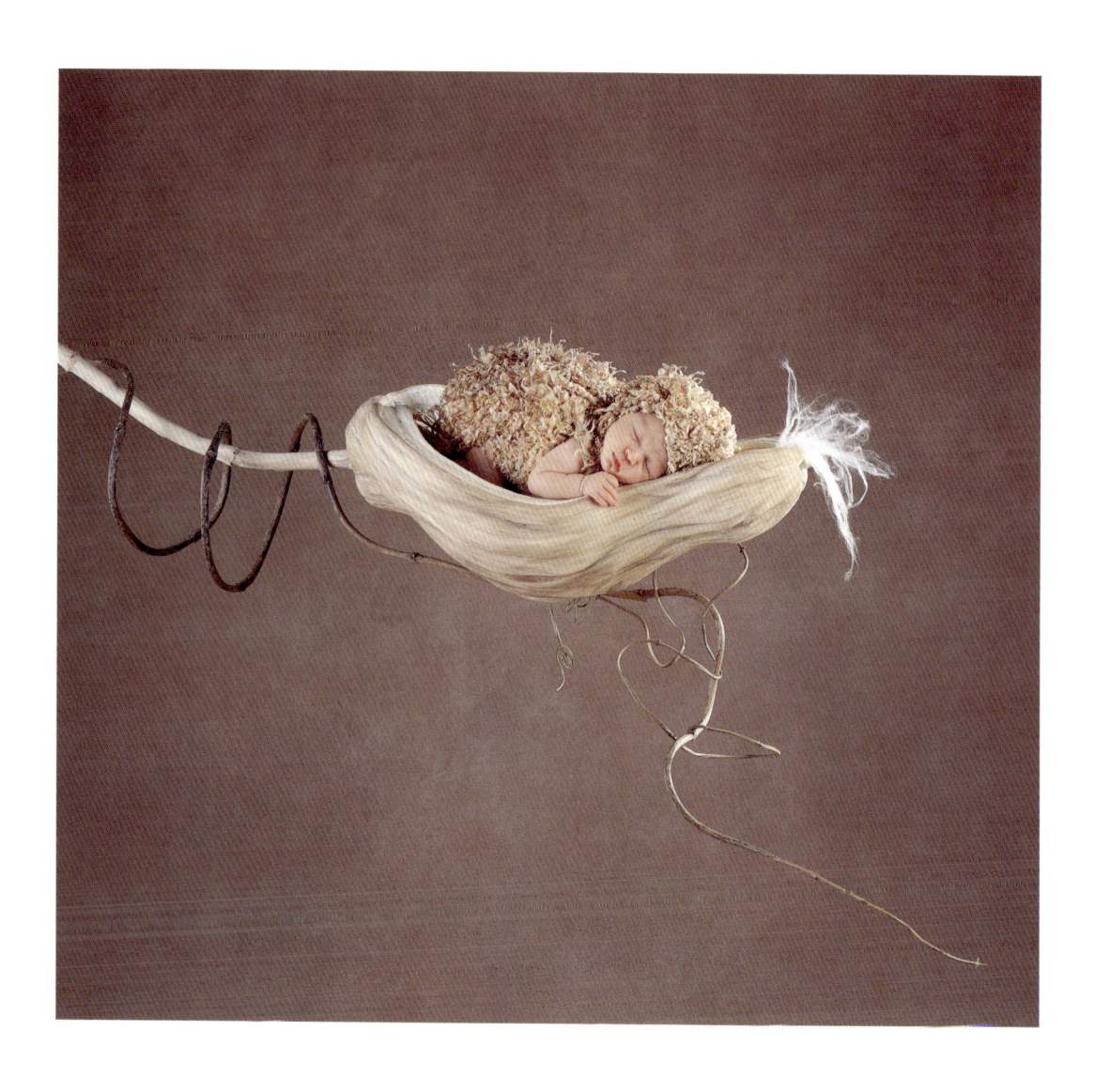

*Things I most
enjoy doing
for myself*

*I take time for
myself by*

- HOPES AND DREAMS -

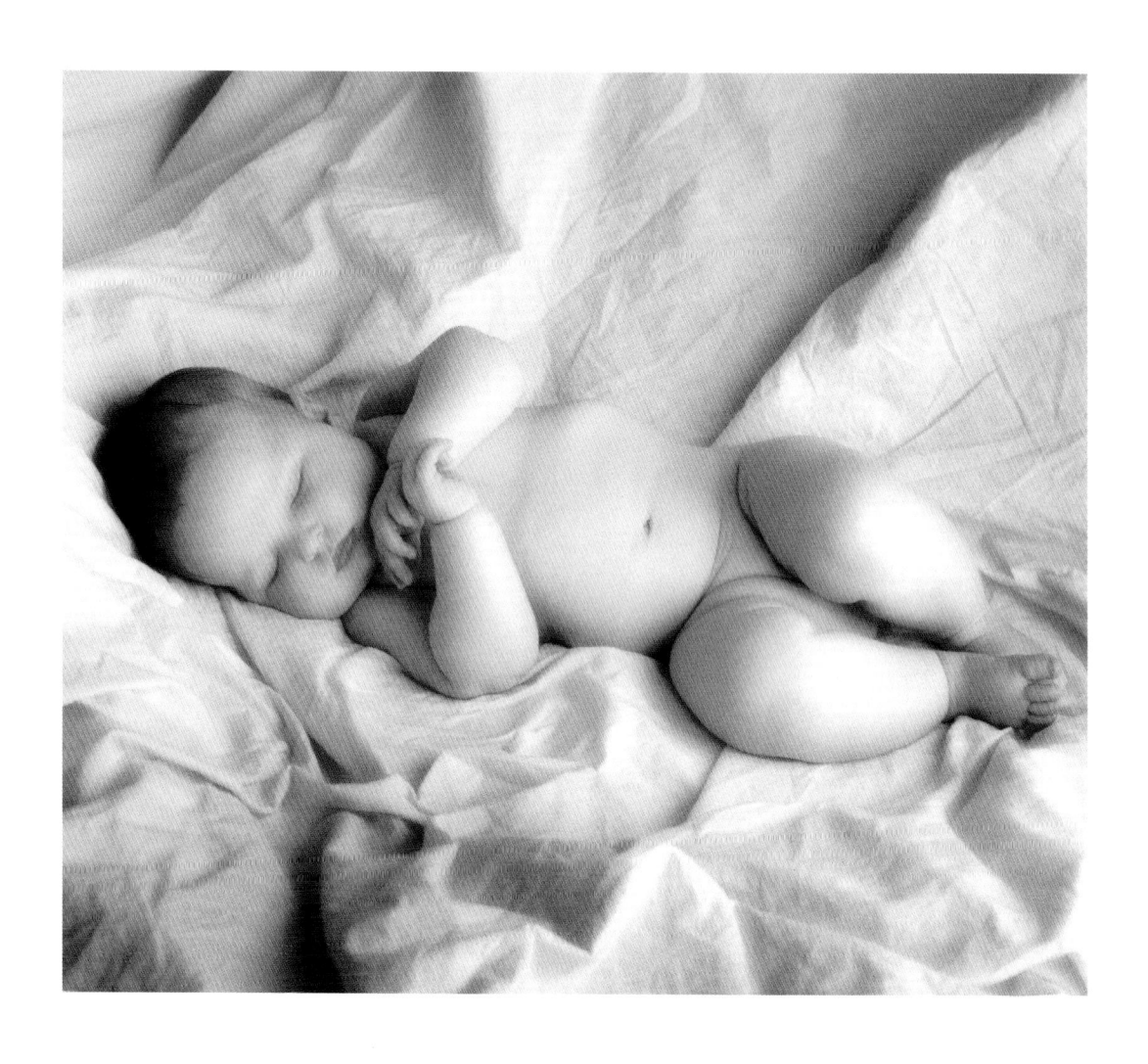

*What I most
wish for
my baby*

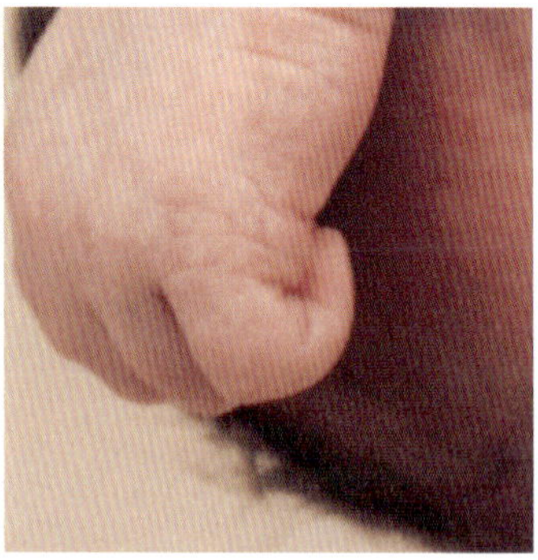

The Final
THREE MONTHS

The Final
THREE MONTHS

- THE HOME STRETCH -

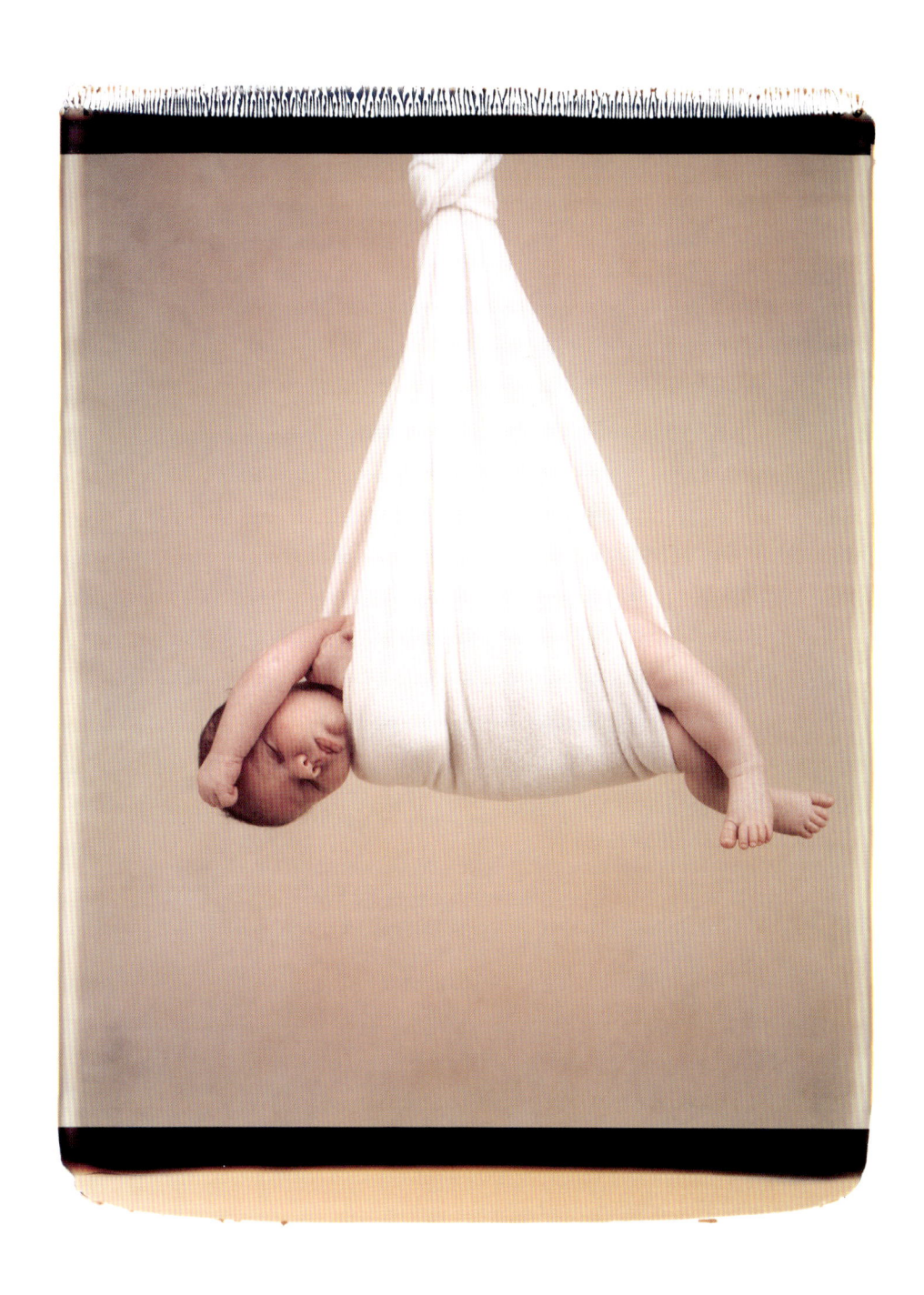

- THE HOME STRETCH -

What I am really enjoying about being pregnant

But this isn't much fun

- THE HOME STRETCH -

Changes I have noticed about my body

- THE HOME STRETCH -

I am excited about

I am feeling anxious about

- THE HOME STRETCH -

Dreams I have been having

What I think they might mean

- ABOUT MY BABY -

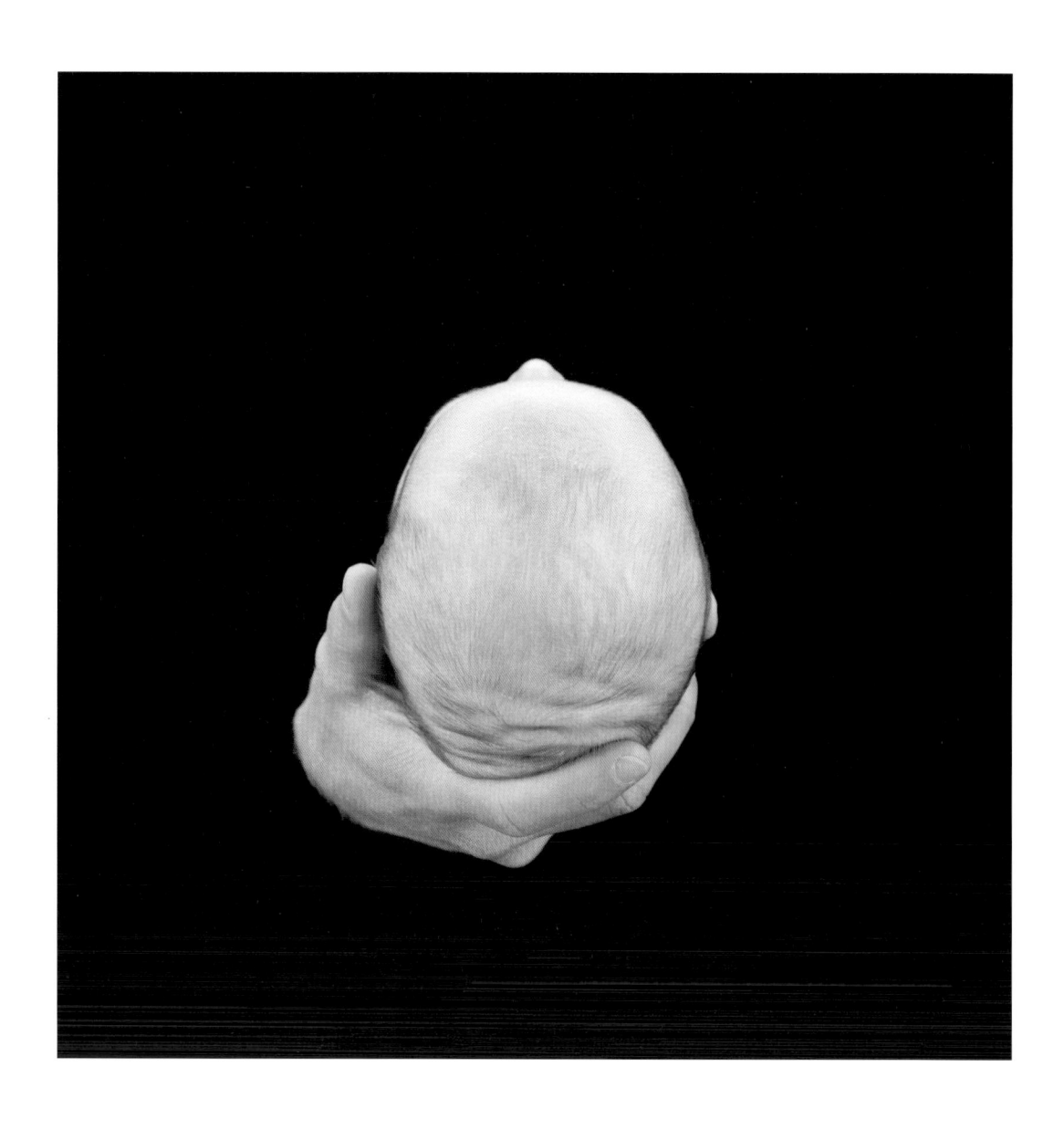

*My baby is
most active*

- ABOUT MY BABY -

My baby seems to respond to

- ABOUT MY BABY -

*Special things
I enjoy doing
for my baby*

- THIS TIME -

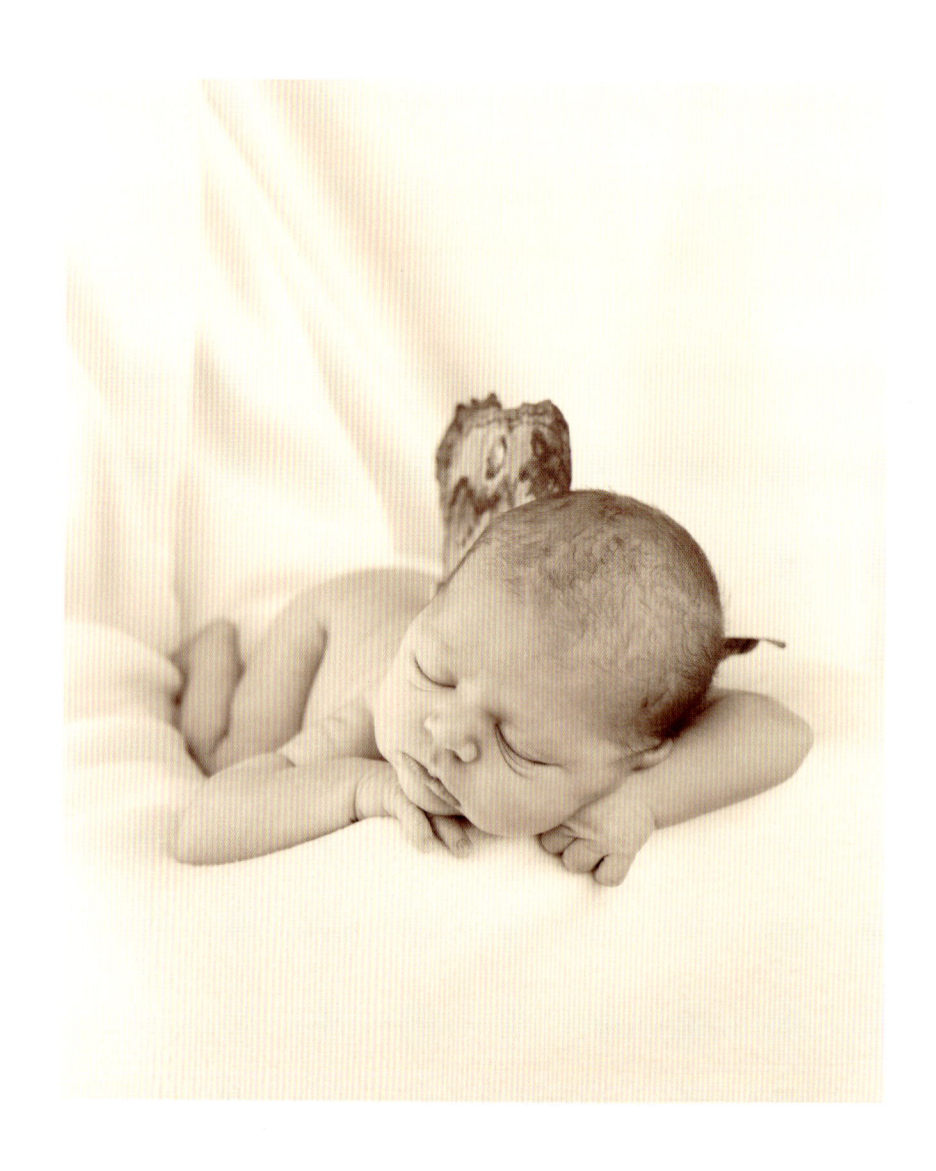

I feel being pregnant this time is either different, or the same, because

- NAMES -

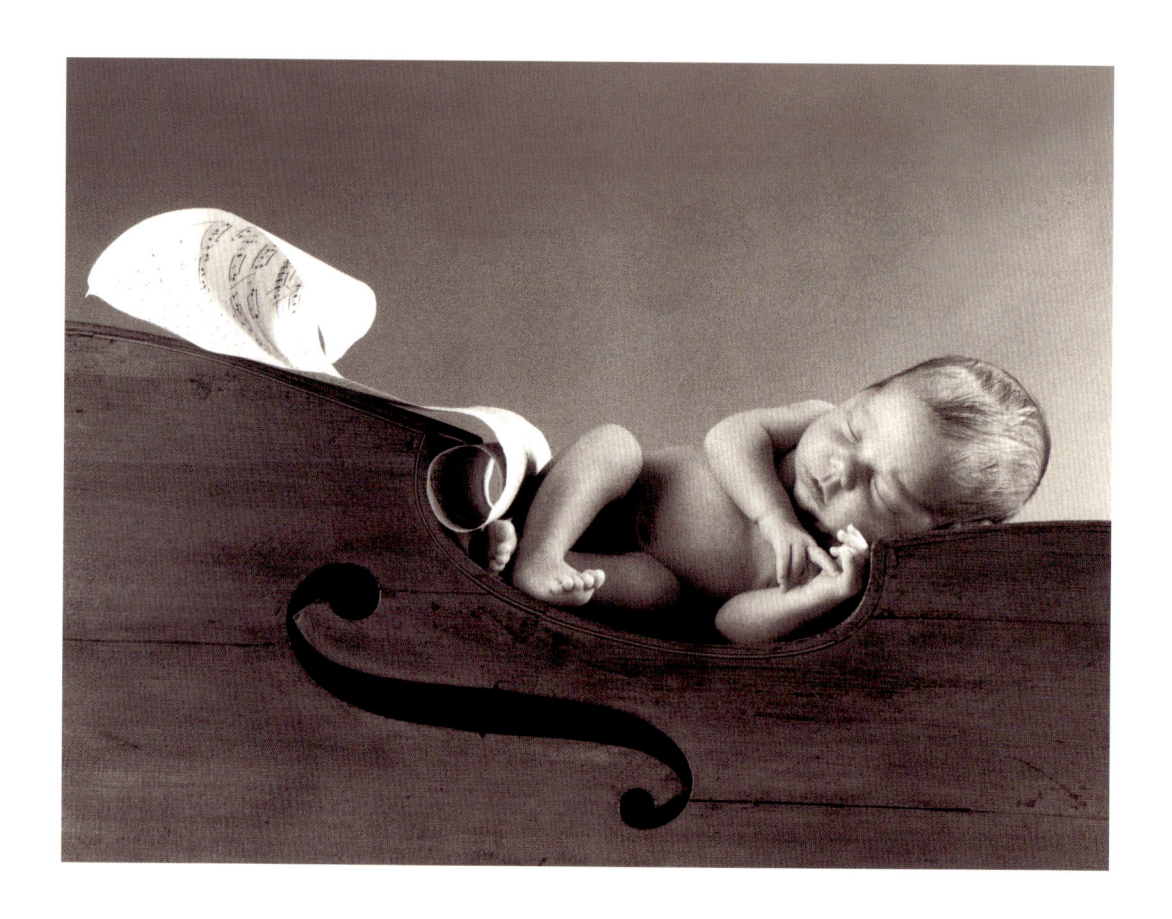

Names I am thinking about for my baby

Boys

Girls

Pet names I have for my baby

- BEST GUESSES -

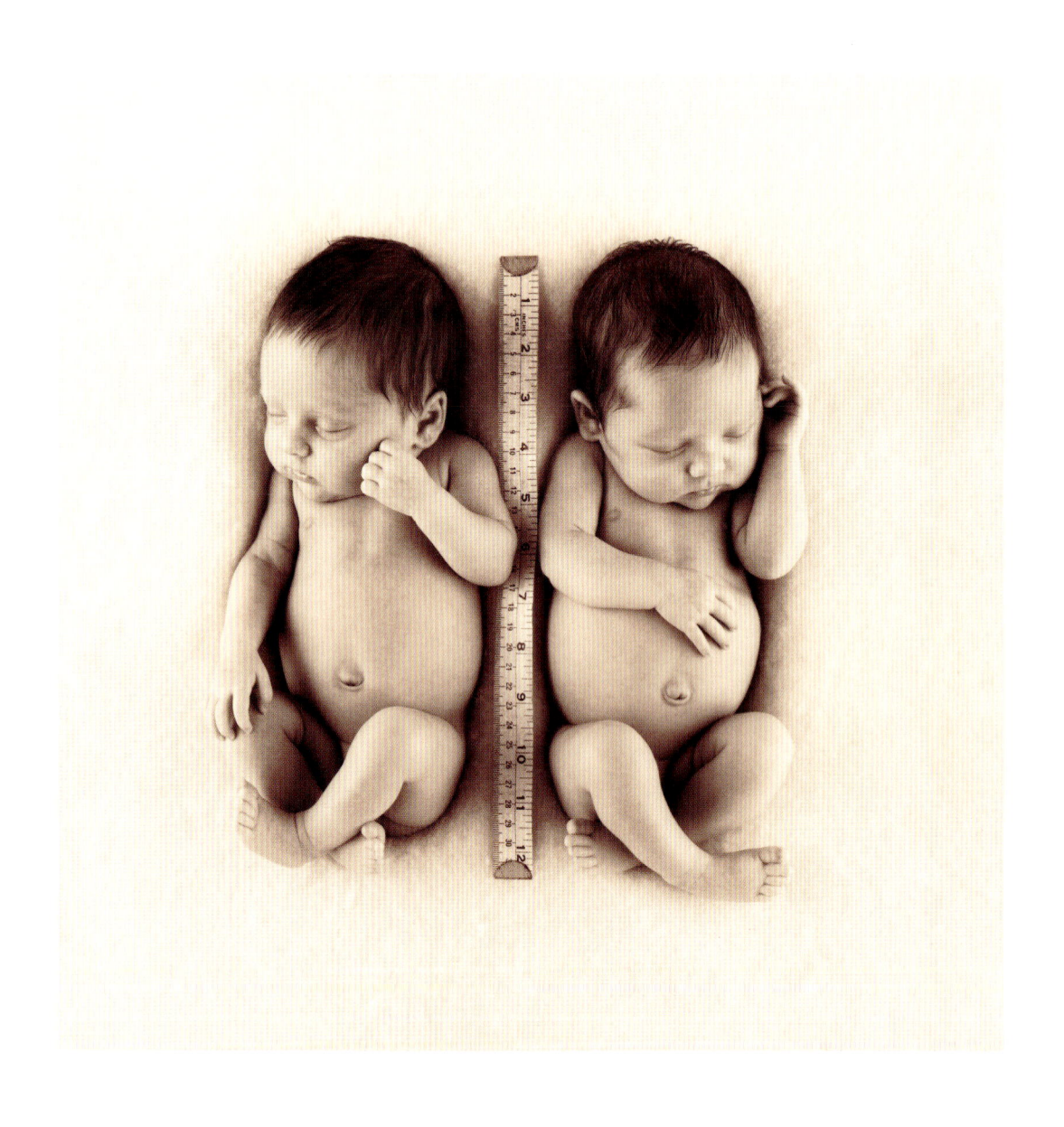

People's comments regarding the likely sex of the baby

My own feelings about the sex of my baby

- FOR THE BABY -

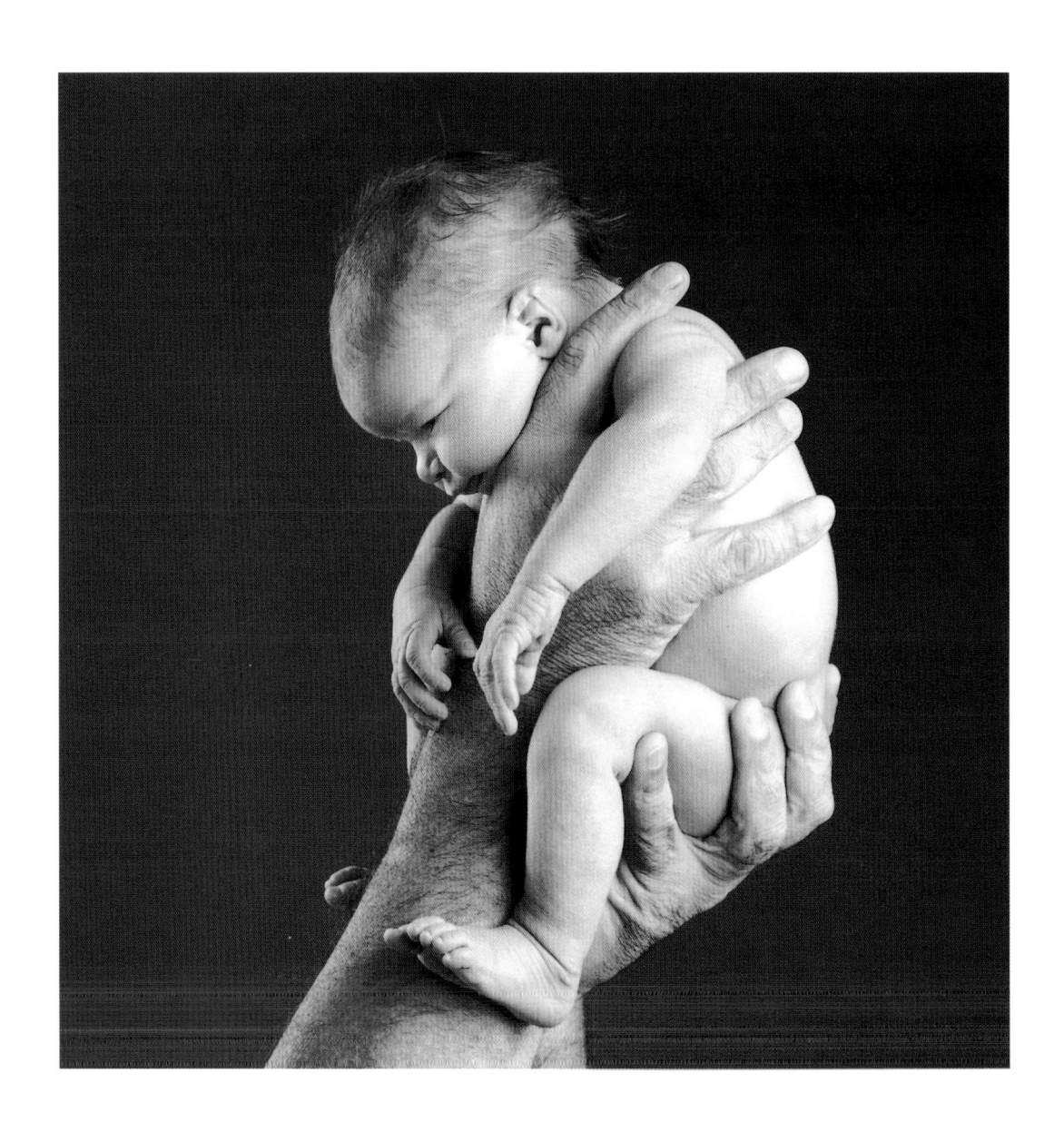

*Special things
I have for
this baby*

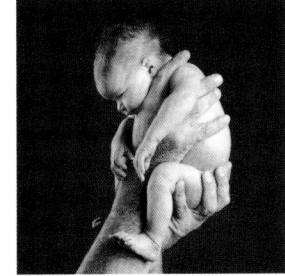

- GIFTS I HAVE RECEIVED -

Gifts I have received . . . from

- FAVORITE CLOTHES -

My favorite piece of clothing is . . . because

- LOOKING BACK -

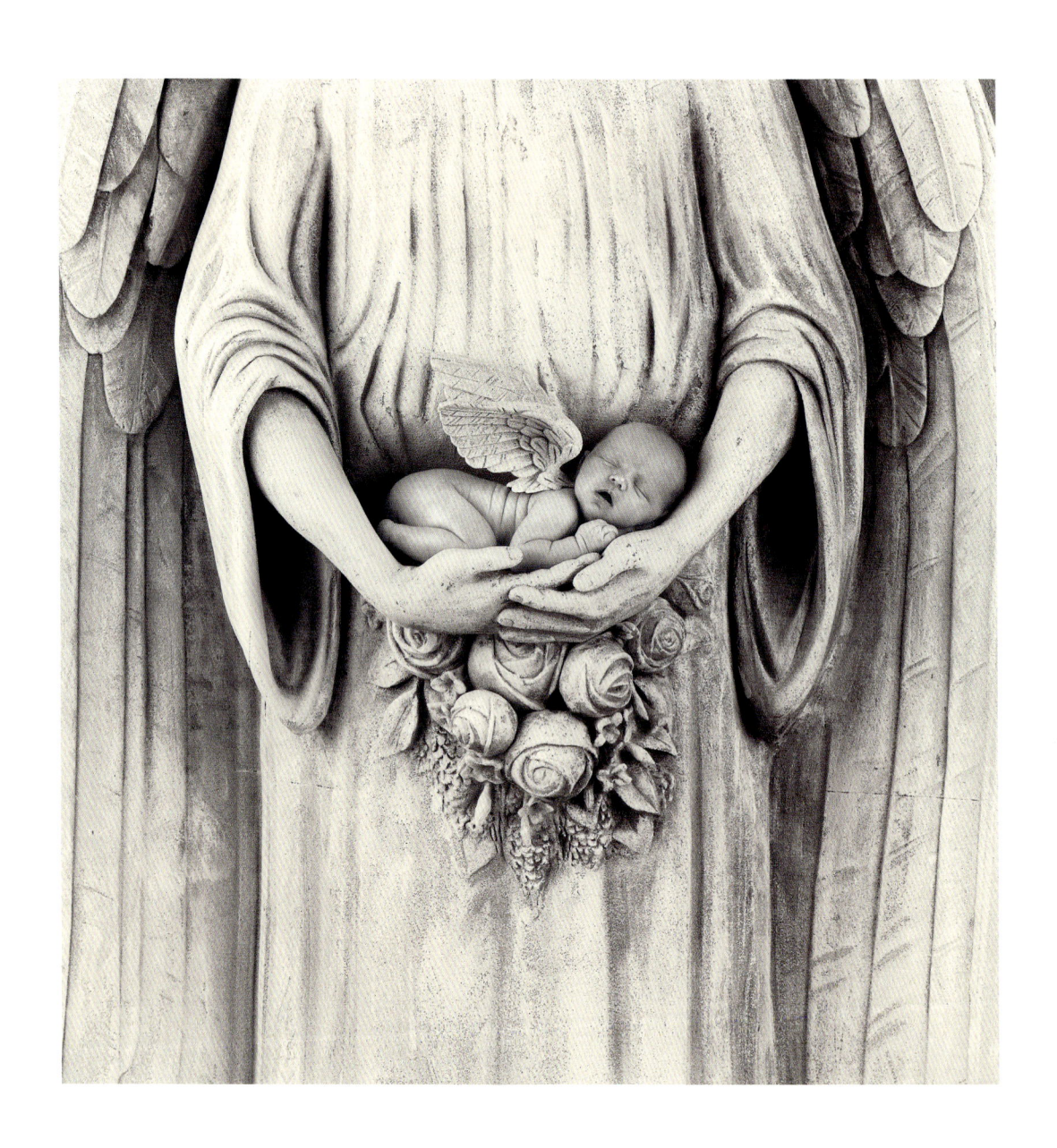

*The best
thing about
being pregnant
has been*

- LOOKING BACK -

The worst thing about being pregnant has been

- LOOKING BACK -

Being pregnant has taught me

I have had great support from

- ANOTHER SPECIAL NOTE TO MY BABY -

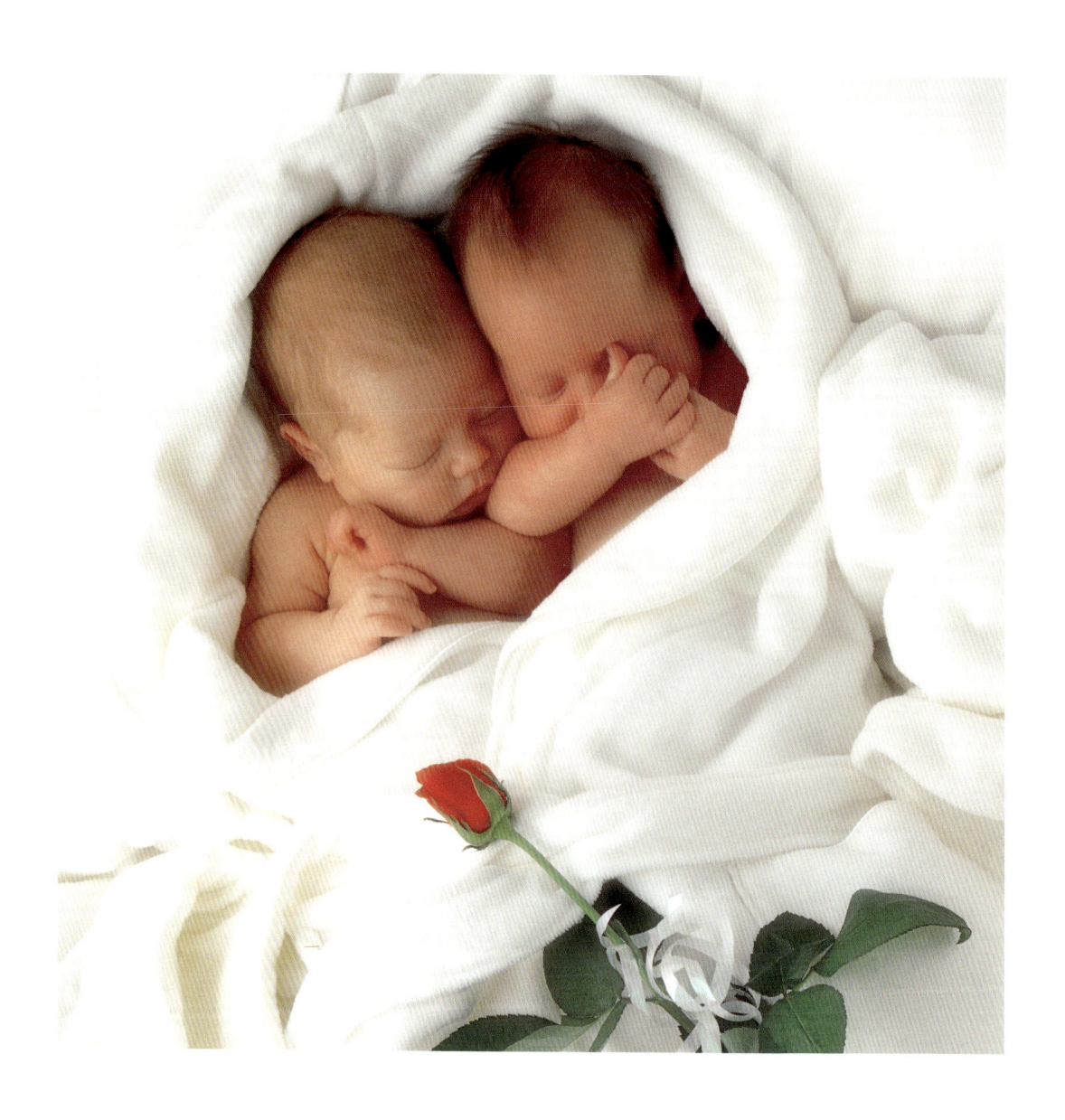

I have been thinking about

I would like you to know

- LOOKING FORWARD -

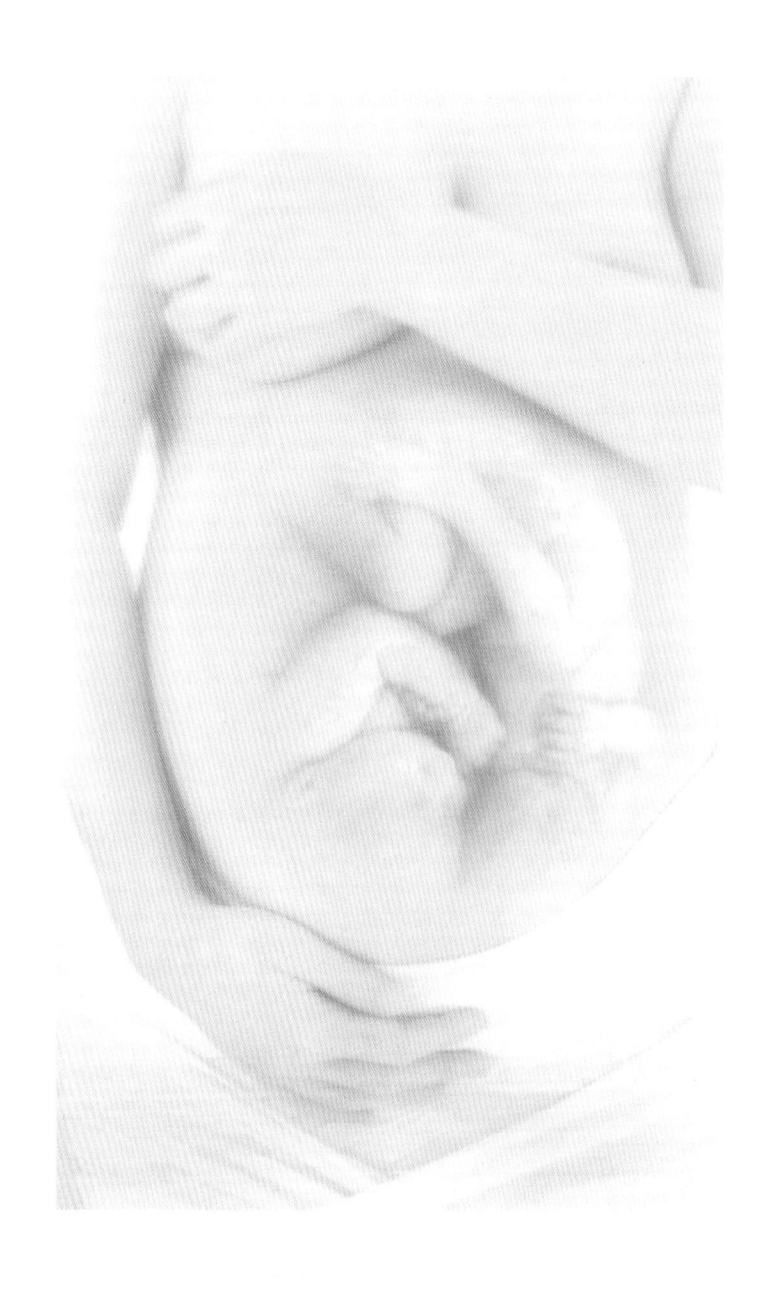

My thoughts about giving birth

- LOOKING FORWARD -

Who I want to support me at the birth

Who else I would like to be with me to share the experience

- LOOKING FORWARD -

I am excited about

I feel anxious about

- BITS & PIECES -

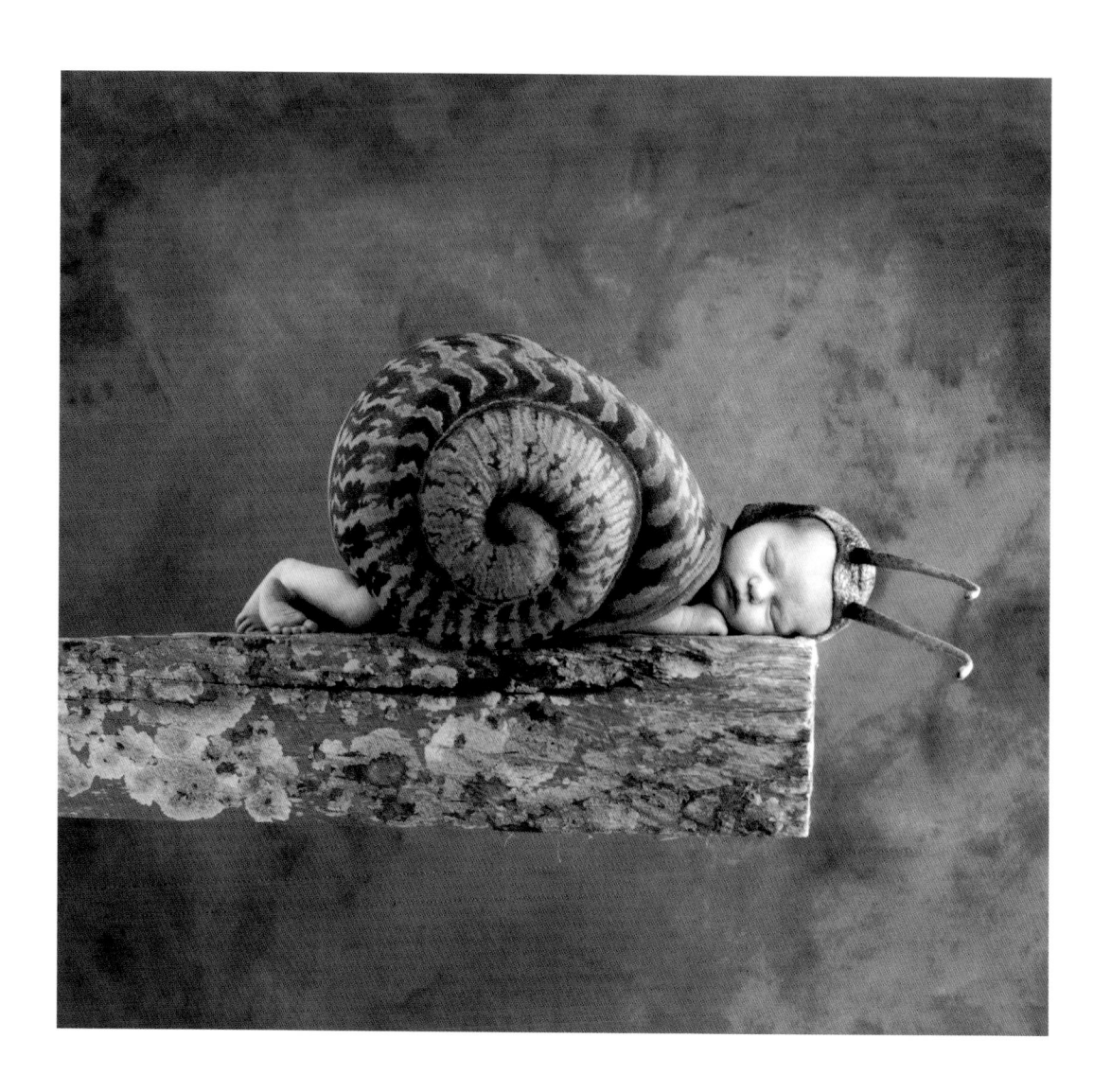

*Special things
I would like to
have with me
at the birth*

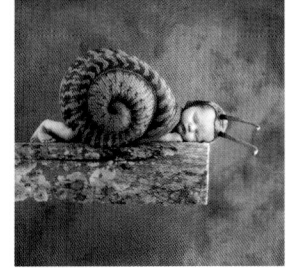

- THE BIRTH OF MY BABY -

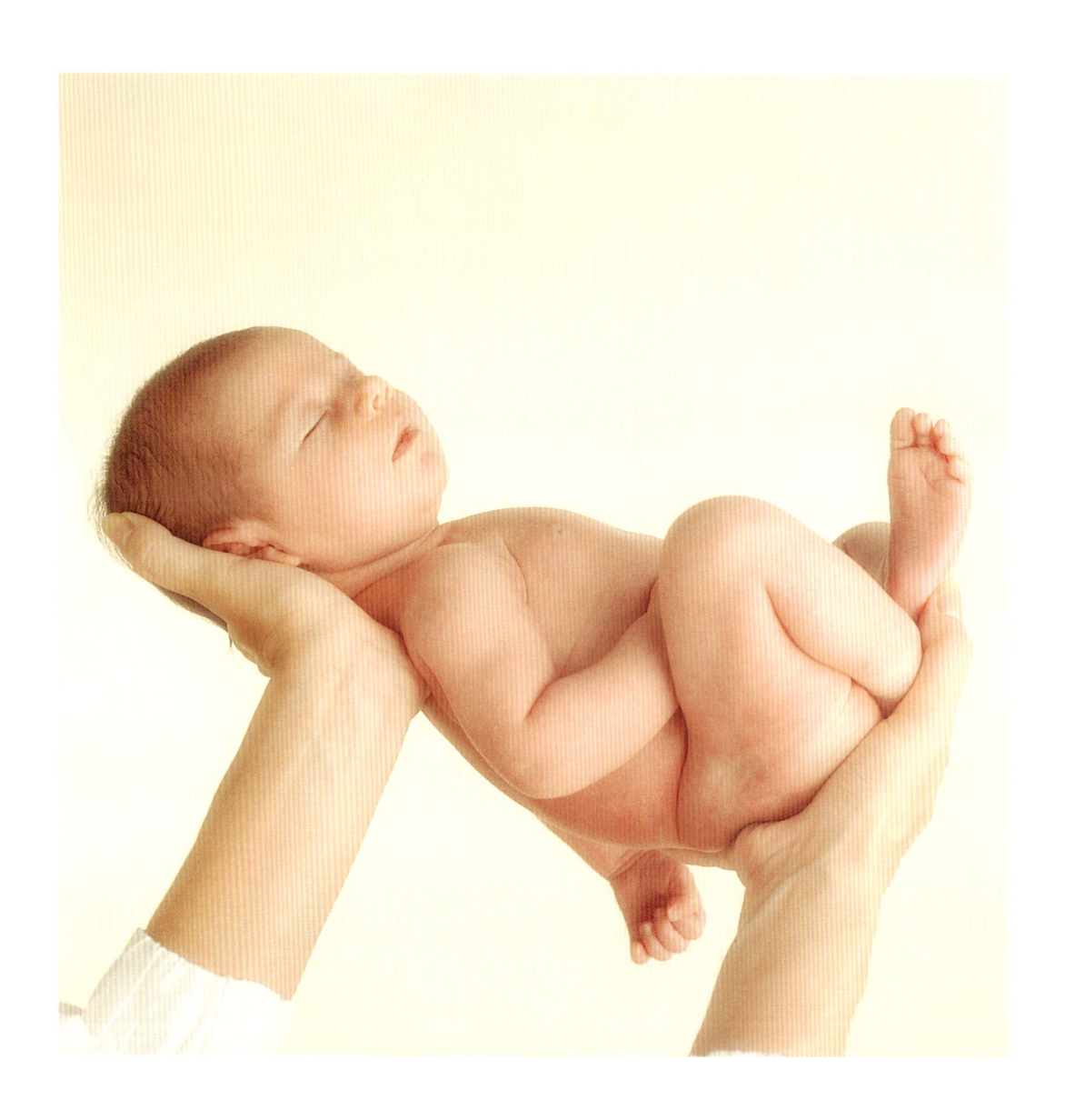

*I knew I was
in labor
because*

Where I was

Date and time

- THE BIRTH -

Who was with me at the birth

- THE BIRTH -

Comments about the labor

- FIRST IMPRESSIONS -

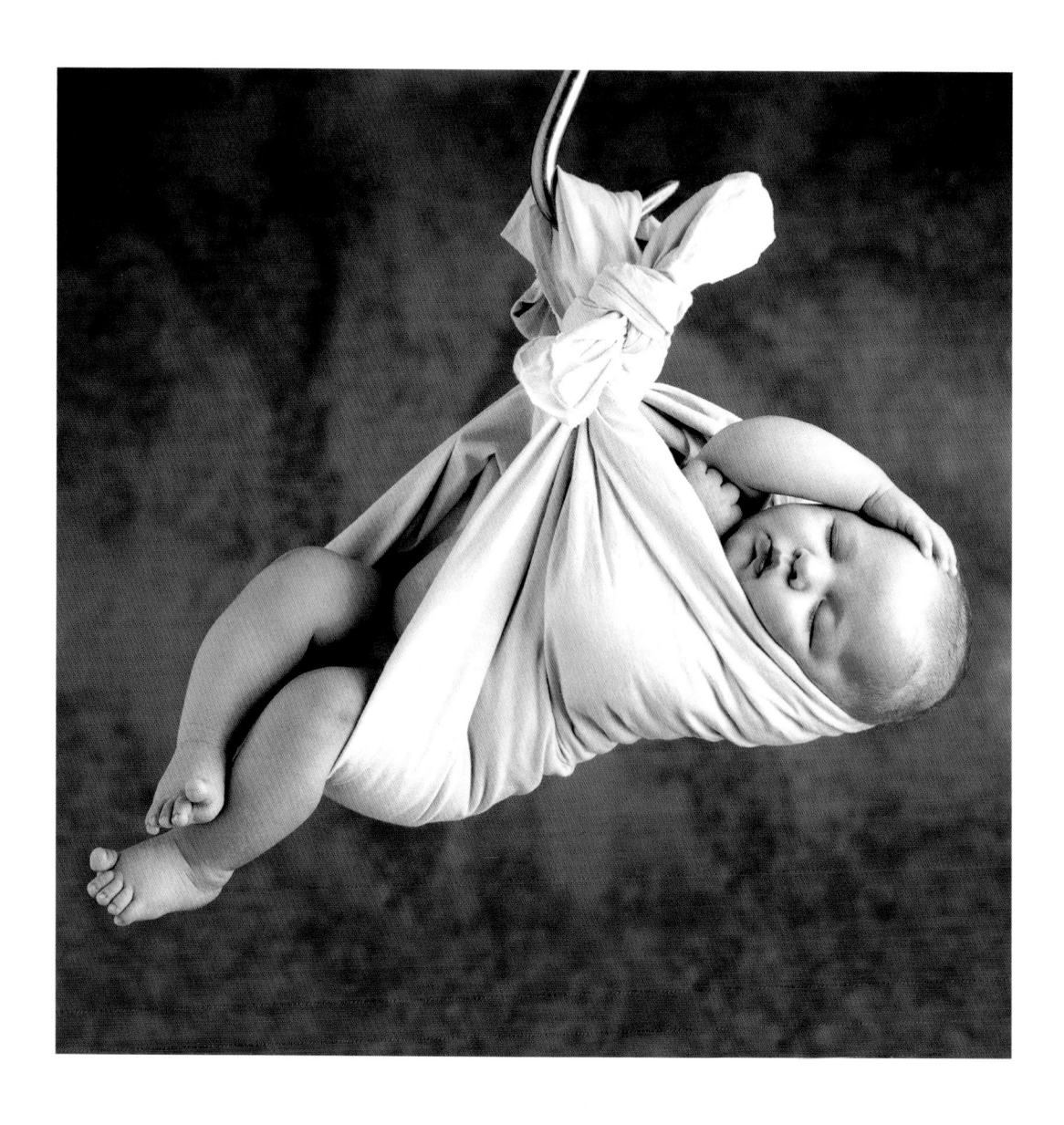

Who cried first

My first words to my baby

- FIRST IMPRESSIONS -

My first thoughts and feelings when my baby was born

Who my baby looks most like

- FIRST IMPRESSIONS -

My biggest surprise about giving birth

- A SPECIAL NOTE TO ME -

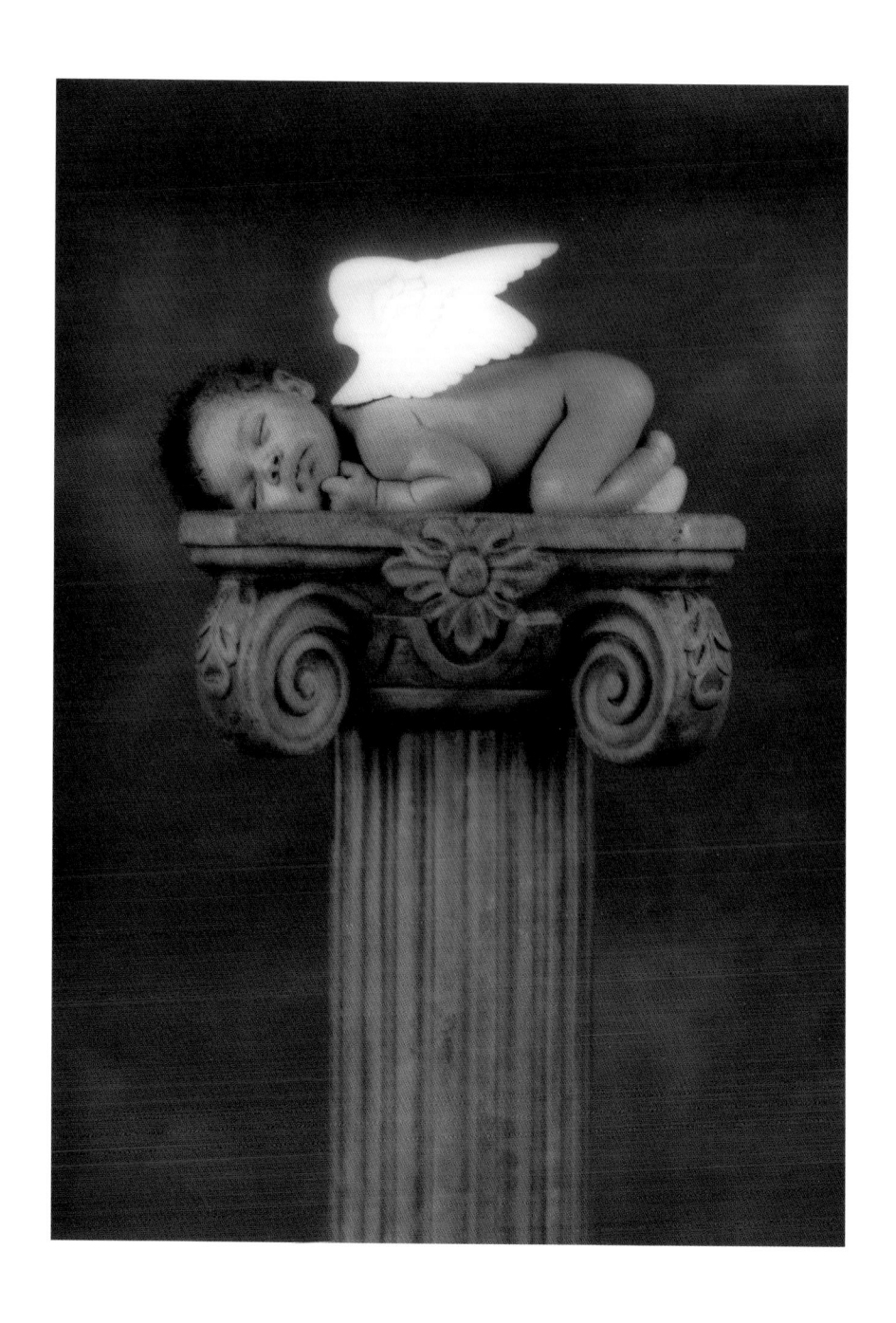

*I feel really
proud of
myself because*

- JUST ME -

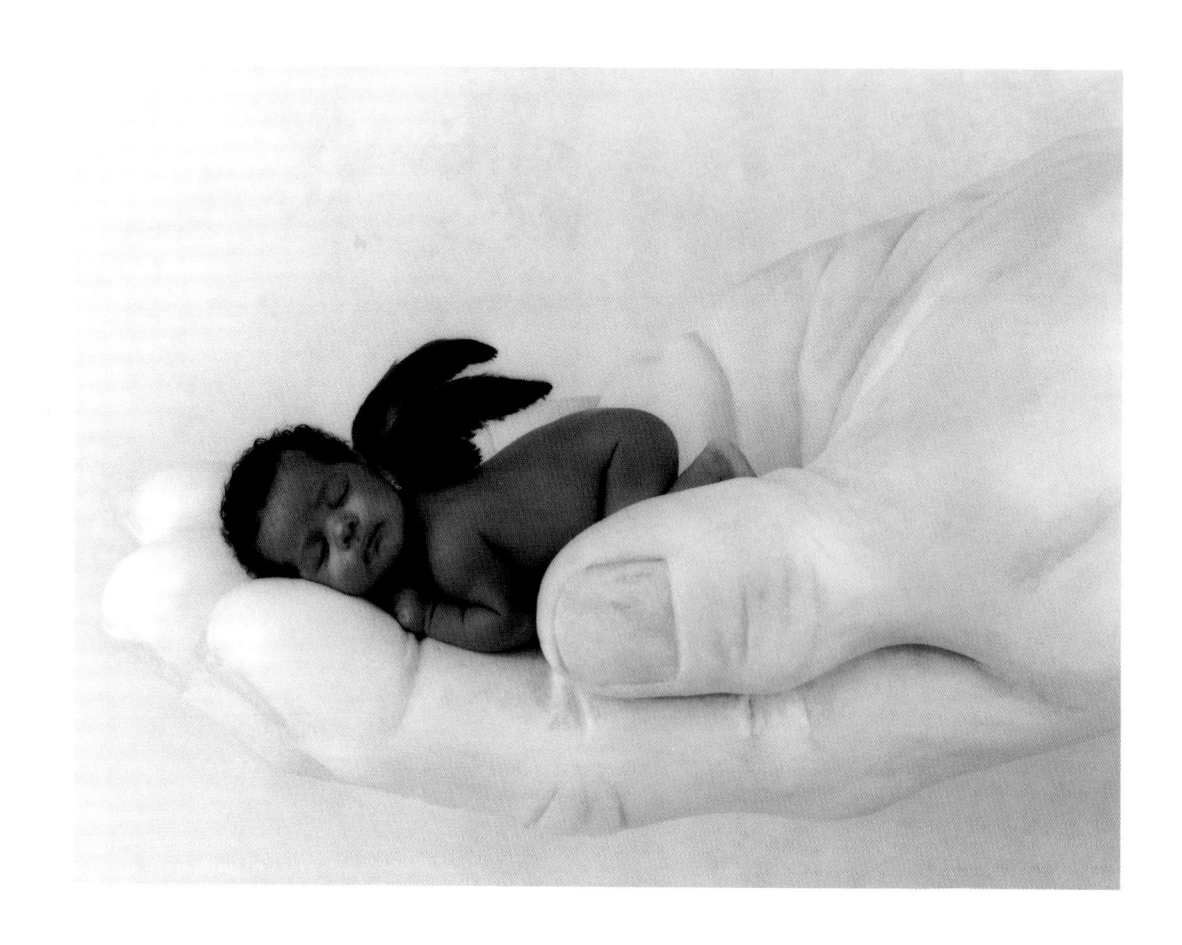

The best thing about not being pregnant

Anything I miss about being pregnant

A NOTE TO OTHERS -

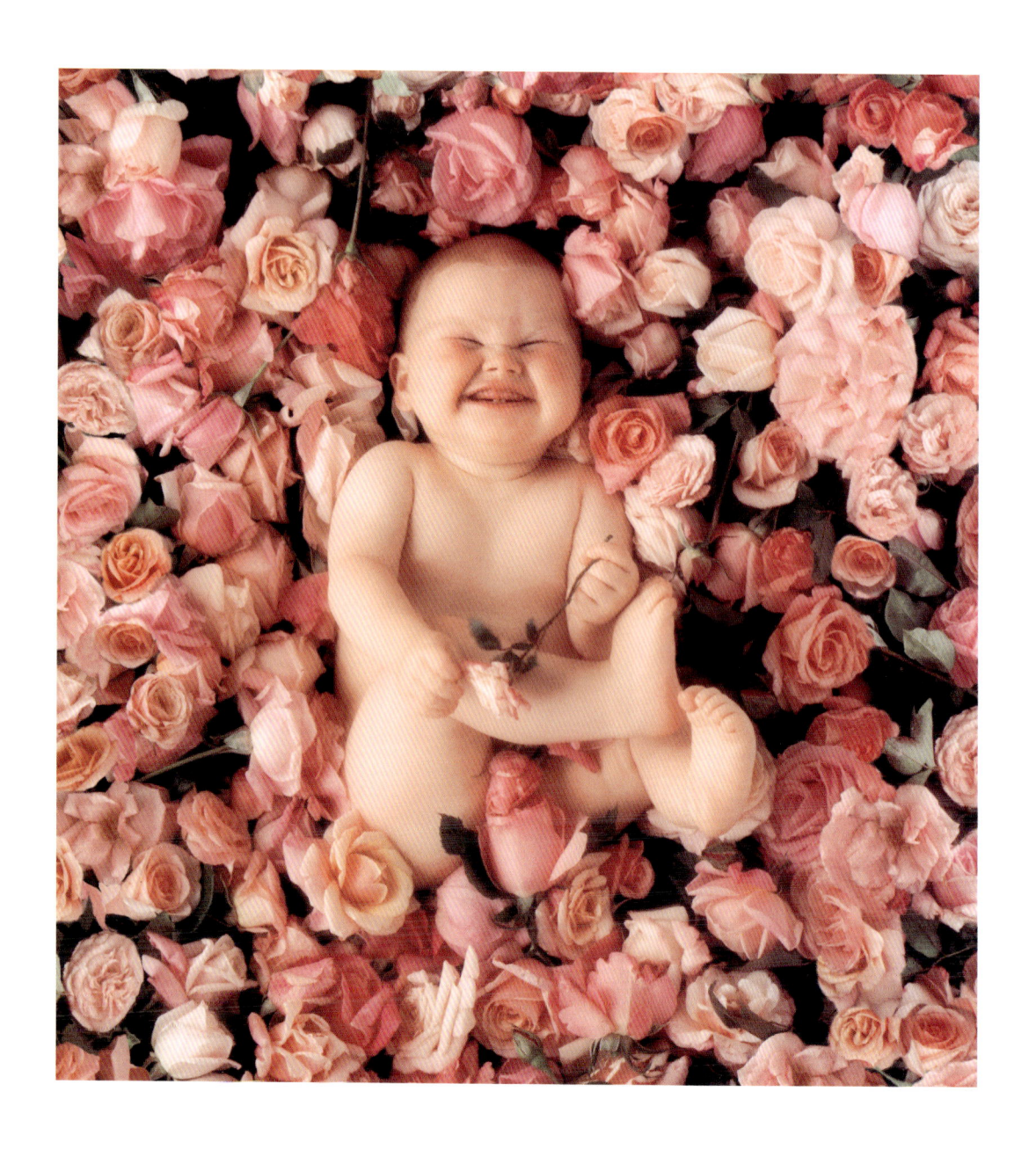

The single best piece of advice I could give to other pregnant women

ANNE GEDDES

ISBN 0-8362-1913-9

© 1999 Anne Geddes

Published in 1999 by Photogenique Publishers
(a division of Hodder Moa Beckett)
Studio 3.16, Axis Building, 1 Cleveland Rd, Parnell
Auckland, New Zealand

First Canadian edition published in 1999 by Andrews McMeel Publishing,
4520 Main Street, Kansas City, MO 64111-7701

Designed by Lucy Richardson
Produced by Kel Geddes
Text researched by Bridget Gordon
Color Separations by MH Group

Printed by Midas Printing Limited, Hong Kong

All rights reserved. No part of this publication may be reproduced
(except brief passages for the purpose of a review),
stored in a retrieval system or transmitted in any form by any means,
electronic, mechanical, photocopying, recording or otherwise,
without the prior written permission of the publisher.

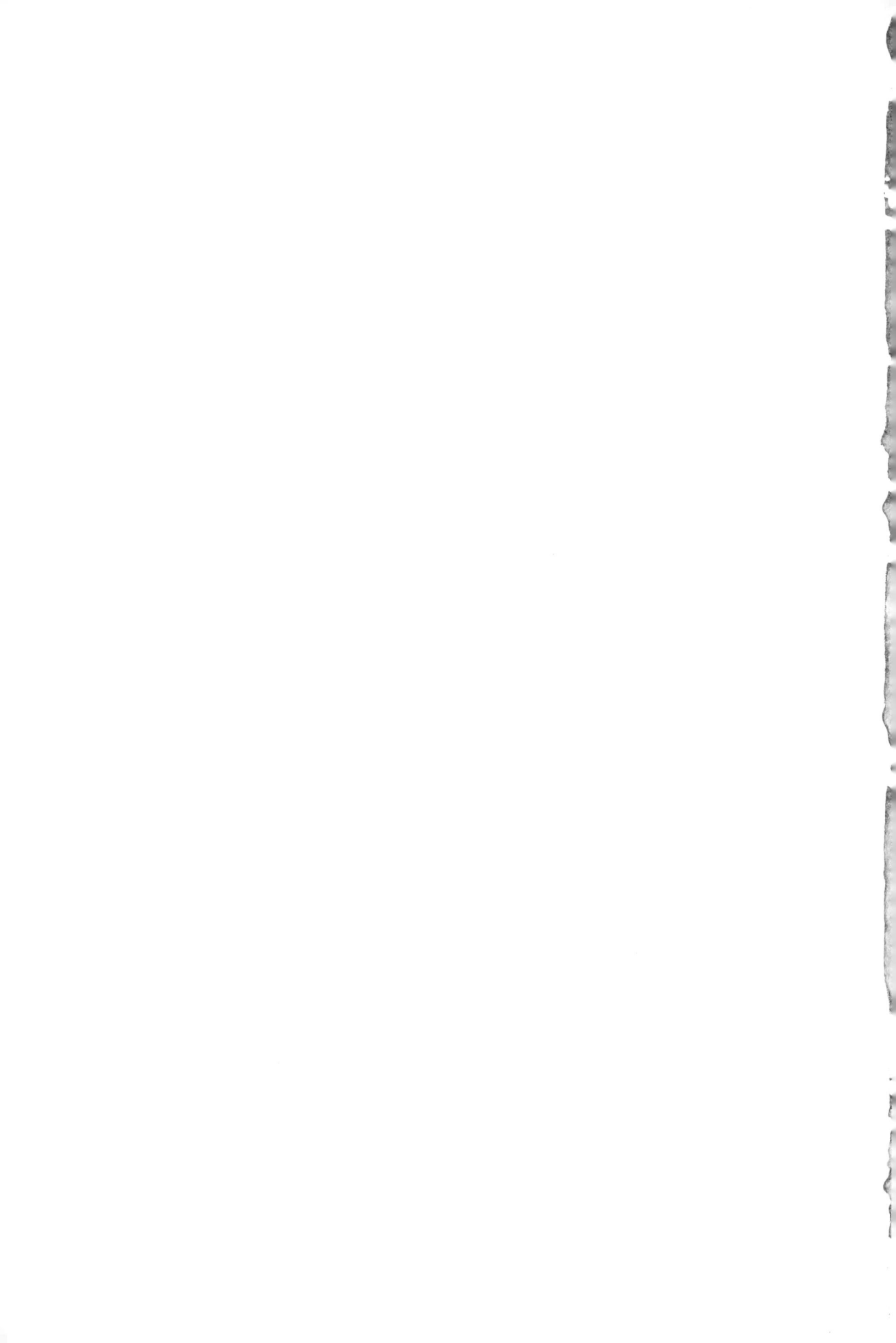